Y0-ABS-205

Y͟   ͟nts

Edited by Jerald D. Hawkins, EdD, ATC, FACSM

ISBN No. 0944183093
Library of Congress No. 91-068118

Published by:
Professional Reports Corporation
4571 Stephen Circle, N.W.
Canton, Ohio 44718-3629

Printed by:
Professional Printing Services
a Division of Professional Reports Corporation
4571 Stephen Circle, N.W.
Canton, Ohio 44718-3629

Cover design by:
Laurance C. Herbert

Distributed by:
Professional Reports Corporation
4571 Stephen Circle, N.W.
Canton, Ohio 44718-3629

Table of Contents

This book is dedicated to memory of

Coach Roy Harmon

– respected coach, beloved teacher,
and Christian gentleman who taught me
that winning is neither everything nor the only thing.

JDH

Publisher's Notice

This publication is written and published to provide accurate and authoritative information relevant to the subject matter presented. It is published and sold with the understanding that the authors and publisher are not engaged in rendering legal, medical, or other professional services by reason of their authorship or publication of this work. If legal, medical or other expert assistance is required, the services of competent professional persons should be sought. Moreover, in the field of coaching, athletic training and sports medicine, the services of such competent professionals must be obtained.

Adapted from a Declaration of Principles of the American Bar Association and a Committee of Publishers and Associations.

Professional Reports Corporation
4571 Stephen Circle, N.W.
Canton, Ohio 44718-3629
(800) 336-0083

Contributing Authors

Dr. Herb Appenzeller is Jefferson-Pilot Professor of Sport Management at Guilford College, and Executive Director of the Sport Studies Foundation. An eminent authority in sport management and sport law, he is co-author of **FROM THE GYM TO THE JURY** newsletter, and author of numerous books and articles on sport management and sport law.

Dr. Mark Bartz is in private family medicine practice with, and co-founder of the Family Physicians of Greenwood, Greenwood, South Carolina. He is a Diplomate of the American Academy of Family Practice.

Dr. John Bourgeois is a practicing ophthalmologist at the Charlotte Eye, Ear, Nose, and Throat Associates. He is a member of Alpha Omega Alpha medical honor society and the Association for Research in Vision and Ophthalmology.

Dr. Ted Burnett is in private dental practice in Winston-Salem, North Carolina. A past-president of the Gate City Dental Study Club, he is a Fellow in the Academy of General Dentistry, and a member of the American Society of Dentistry for Children.

Dr. Joe Chandler is Professor and Chairman of the Division of Physical Education and Exercise Studies at Lander College, Greenwood, South Carolina. He is a Fellow in the American College of Sports Medicine and a South Carolina Certified Athletic Trainer. He has taught human anatomy and physiology for eighteen years. He is the author of numerous publications on physical fitness, anatomy and physiology, and exercise science.

Dr. Dan Garfinkel is a physician with the Urgent Medical Care Center, Greensboro, North Carolina. A member of the American Academy of Sports Physicians, he is the author of numerous publications on psychology and youth sports. He is team physician for several area high schools, and for the Greensboro Hornets professional baseball club.

Mrs. Renee Garfinkel is a graduate of Hunter College with a degree in psychology. A volunteer speaker and consultant on child abuse, she has many years experience as a "Little League" mother and advocate of youth sports programs.

Dr. Stan Grosshandler is a member of the Raleigh Pain Clinic, and Clinical Associate Professor of Anesthesiology at the University of North Carolina, Chapel Hill, North Carolina. He is an authority on sports history and author of numerous publications on that subject.

Dr. Bob Gwyther is Associate Professor of Family Medicine in the School of Medicine at the University of North Carolina, Chapel Hill, North Carolina. Director of the Family Practice Center, he is the author of numerous publications.

Dr. John Hall is in private dermatology practice in Greensboro, North Carolina. A Clinical Associate Professor at the University of North Carolina, Chapel Hill, North Carolina, he is on the Board of Directors of the North American Clinical Dermatologic Society, and author of numerous publications on acne and other skin infections.

Dr. Jerry Hawkins is Professor, Coordinator of Exercise Studies, and Director of Sports Medicine Services at Lander College, Greenwood, South Carolina. A Fellow in the American College of Sports Medicine, a National Athletic Trainers' Association Certified Athletic Trainer, and a South Carolina Certified Athletic Trainer, he has had numerous international sports medicine appointments including the Junior Luge World Championships and Goodwill Games. He is author of numerous publications on sports medicine, physical fitness and exercise science.

Dr. John King is in private orthopaedic practice with the Greenwood Orthopaedic Clinic, Greenwood, South Carolina. A candidate member of the American Academy of Orthopaedic Surgery, he is a member of the Lander College Sports Medicine Services Team.

Dr. Jim Manly is former team physician for North Carolina State University, and is recognized as an authority in the areas of internal and sports medicine.

Dr. J. M. McWhorter is Associate Professor of Neurology at the Bowman Gray School of Medicine, Winston-Salem, North Carolina. A member of the American Association of Neurological Surgeons, he has served as a member of the State Superintendent of Public Instruction Sports Medicine Advisory Commission and is author of numerous publications.

Dr. Gabe Mirkin is in private practice in Silver Springs, Maryland. A widely-recognized authority in sports medicine, he is a nationally-syndicated columnist, television broadcaster and talk show host. He is author of numerous publications including The Sports Medicine Book.

Dr. Louie Patsevouras is in private practice in plastic and reconstructive surgery in Greensboro, North Carolina. He is a member of the Academy of Otolaryngology-Head and Neck Surgery and the American Academy of Facial, Plastic, and Reconstructive Surgery.

Dr. Mona Shangold is Associate Professor and Director of the Sports Gynecology and Woman's Life Cycle Center at Hahnemann University, Philadelphia, Pennsylvania. An eminent authority in the field of sport gynecology, she is a Fellow in the American College of Sports Medicine and a United States Olympic Committee Sports Medicine Research Associate. She is a contributing editor to several well-known publications and author of numerous publications on sport gynecology.

Dr. Bruce Shields is Professor of Ophthalmology at Duke University, Durham, North Carolina. Past president of the North Carolina Ophthalmological Society and committee chairman of the National Society to Prevent Blindness, he was recipient of the Davison Award for Excellence in Teaching at the Duke University Medical School.

Dr. Tom Stevens is Associate Professor of Physical Education and Exercise Studies at Lander College, Greenwood, South Carolina. A certified Coaching Education Instructor with the American Coaching Effectiveness Program, he is Director of Coaching Education at Lander College.

Dr. Tim Taft is Professor of Orthopaedics at the University of North Carolina Medical School, Chapel Hill, North Carolina. The author of numerous publications, he is team orthopaedist for the University of North Carolina. He has extensive experience in international sports medicine, having been named team physician for the United States Pan American Games Team, the United States World University Games Team and the United States Olympic Team.

Foreword

Youth sports have become an integral and vital aspect of American society. Opportunities within a given community for participation in youth sports have grown to include more children, and to provide a wider variety of sport experiences. Central to the success of the various programs that have developed has been, and continues to be the involvement of volunteer coaches and parents. Further, a successful program is one in which its volunteer coaches have received specialized training on coaching techniques, and in the legal, scientific, and medical foundations of the sport. Likewise, an informed and educated parent contributes to the overall health of the program and its young athletes.

Coaches and parents often have questions and concerns relating to various aspects of youth sports, but are frequently faced with a situation in which they do not know who to ask, or where to go for answers. Typical questions might include the following:

"What is my legal liability as a coach?"

"What should my athletes or my children be eating to best prepare for their sport?"

"Should I be concerned about my athletes' or my children's weight?"

"How can I best condition my athletes or my child for their sport? Should I encourage distance running? Strength training?"

"How extensive a medical examination should be required for participation in any given sport?"

"What if one of my athletes or my children is injured? What care should be given? Who should we see? How can we be referred to a specialist?"

"Who should determine when an injured child can safely return to participation, and on what basis should this decision be made?"

The realization that coaches and parents do have a number of important questions and concerns that are not easily answered was the driving force for the development of this book.

This book was written by a group of experts in sport law, sports medicine, and sports science, to provide the volunteer coach and the parent with basic information relating to each of their specialties. Each of the experts was given the challenge of writing a brief overview of his/her area of specialization, with information which is practical and interesting. Translating legal, medical, and scientific information into a readable and practical format is the mark of a successful book of this type. The editor and contributing authors are to be congratulated on hitting the mark!

The editor and authors have worked hard to provide an informative and practical document. Now, the ball is in your court! By reading and using this book, your responsibilities as a youth sports coach and/or parent should be made easier and more enjoyable.

Jack H. Wilmore, PhD, FACSM
Margie Gurley Seay Centennial Professor
Department of Kinesiology and Health Education
The University of Texas at Austin

Chapter I

Legal Aspects

Herbert T. Appenzeller and Jerald D. Hawkins

No one wants the young athlete to be injured. In sports activities, however, there is always the possibility of injury no matter how carefully proper procedures are observed. In like manner, no one wants to be a defendant in a lawsuit. Today there is unprecedented interest in youth sports, and this all-time high rate of participation is accompanied by a record number of sports-related lawsuits.

Youth Sports and Litigation

The fact that an injury occurs does not necessarily mean that the coach is negligent or liable for damages, or that he/she will be sued as a result of the injury. In our legal system, there are no definite criteria for determining specifically what is and is not negligent behavior, since each case stands on its own merit.

While the threat of expensive litigation is very real, youth sport personnel have enjoyed relatively rare immunity from suit. This probably results from the fact that most people believe that the majority of youth sports coaches and physicians volunteer their services for altruistic reasons rather than financial gain. Regarding the lack of litigation against the amateur team physician when compared to the professional team physician, Michael Gallagher, an Ohio attorney has commented:

"I think it is because a competitive sports team physician holds a unique position in the eyes, and if you will, the hearts of our athletes to whom he ministers and, indeed, of their parents as well. Team physicians are not rewarded economically; their primary interest is in helping youngsters. This awareness on the part of the athletes and their parents plays a large part in protecting the physician from litigation."

In the above statement, the term "volunteer coach" may easily be substituted for the word "physician", which may explain the small number of lawsuits against volunteer coaches. However, it should not be assumed that there cannot or will not be litigation against the volunteer coach. The threat of litigation is ever present, and can develop quickly without warning. Therefore, every youth sports coach and/or volunteer worker should make every effort possible to avoid situations which are likely to result in litigation.

Liability of Youth Sports Coaches

Youth sports volunteers (coaches, physicians, etc.) should not have a false sense of security regarding litigation. Volunteers are liable for their acts of negligence, even when they do not receive compensation for their services unless particular state laws provide immunity to such volunteers.

Because of the increase in sports-related lawsuits in the 1980s, many states have passed legislation designed to protect volunteer coaches and physicians from liability. Approximately one-half of all state legislatures have enacted statutes which provide immunity for volunteers in nonprofit organizations. There are, however, exclusions to these statutes, and volunteers may be held liable if their conduct constitutes gross negligence or willful and wanton misconduct. Volunteers and officers of all nonprofit organizations should become familiar with statutes in their respective states, and should be aware of specific exclusions which leave them unprotected.

Preventing Injury-Related Litigation

The following recommendations can help prevent situations which may lead to injuries and subsequent litigation:
1. Require a physical examination before the participant engages in the sport.
2. Make certain all equipment fits properly.
3. Inspect all equipment for defects and facilities for hazards.
4. Obtain medical insurance coverage for the youth sport participant and liability insurance for the coach and physician.
5. Adopt a medical plan for emergency treatment.
6. Assign activities within the participant's range of ability and commensurate with his/her size and physical condition.
7. Prepare the participant gradually for all physical drills, and progress from simple to complex tasks.
8. Warn the participant of all possible dangers inherent in the sport.

9. Adopt a policy regarding injuries. Do not attempt to be a "medical specialist" in judging the physical condition of the participant under your care.
10. Require a physician's medical permission before permitting seriously ill or injured participants to return to normal practice and/or game activity.
11. Avoid moving an injured participant until it is safe to do so.
12. Conduct periodic medical in-service training programs for all volunteer coaches.
13. Maintain an appropriately-stocked athletic first aid kit at all practices and games (see Appendix B).
14. Maintain accurate written records of preparticipation medical examinations, injuries which occur, and the specific care which was given injured athletes under your supervision.

Record-Keeping

One of the most effective tools in the prevention of or defense against injury-related litigation is a written record showing that the injury was carefully documented, and that proper care was given to the injured athlete. In the absence of such records, critical facts may be forgotten, misinterpreted, or distorted, making it difficult for the coach or volunteer worker to refute claims of negligence. Unlike college and professional sports programs, youth sports injury records may be relatively simplified, yet specific. The two most important forms which should be maintained in the administrative office of every youth sports program are 1) the preparticipation medical exam and 2) injury report or incidence forms. It is highly recommended that standardized, custom forms be developed which meet the specific needs of the program.

Preparticipation Medical Exam. Every youth sports participant should undergo a medical examination prior to participation in the youth sports program (see Chapter 8). The results of this examination should be recorded by the attending physician, and should be maintained on file in the administrative office of the youth sports program. An example of a comprehensive medical history and examination form is presented in Appendix C. (Note: Forms presented in Appendix C are provided only as examples. Each program should design and utilize forms which meet the specific needs of that program.)

Injury Report. Every injury should be reported to a coach or volunteer worker at the time it occurs. It then becomes the responsibility of the coach or worker to provide first aid care, notify the injured child's parents, and/or arrange for appropriate medical care. Details concerning how the injury occurred and the manner in which it was managed should be carefully and accurately recorded on an injury report form, copies of which should be maintained on file in the administrative offices of the youth sports program. An example of a comprehensive injury report form is presented in Appendix C.

Insurance and Youth Sports

Many sports organizations obtain insurance in an attempt to reduce the potential for litigation. States often waive immunity to the extent of insurance coverage. It is important that volunteer coaches and physicians know the extent of insurance coverage, and any exclusions in the policy which may pertain to them. Many volunteer coaches obtain liability insurance by adding riders to their homeowners policies, under business pursuits. Once again, the volunteer needs to understand the limits and possible exclusions of such insurance coverage. A policy rider is often inexpensive, and can provide valuable coverage for the volunteer.

In addition to liability insurance, many sports organizations secure blanket accident medical insurance for participants in the program, while others require parental insurance. It is crucial that participants have accident insurance coverage. If insurance coverage is provided by or purchased through the sports organization, care should be taken to ensure that participants and parents understand the specific nature of the coverage.

Sports Participation for the Disabled

Each year, numerous young athletes with a variety of physical disabilities enjoy participation in organized sports. Unfortunately, many organizations still follow the 1976 recommendations of the American Medical Association regarding the disqualification of certain athletes for medical reasons, believing them to be mandated regulations. Individuals with one testicle, one eye, or one kidney are routinely denied the opportunity to participate in sports. Federal law (Public Law 94-142) protects these individuals, and requires organizations (if they receive federal funding) to provide opportunities for participation. Also, the Rehabilitation Act of 1973 and the Americans With Disabilities Act of 1990 extends protection from discrimination to certain participants. It is important that all youth sports organizations support federal law, and extend opportunities for participation to otherwise qualified youngsters with disabilities.

4

Chapter II

Anatomical And Physiological Aspects

Joe V. Chandler

The human body is a complex and fascinating structure of interdependent tissues, organs, and systems. Growth, development, and maturation of the body is brought about by the cooperative effort of genes, hormones, nutrients, and a variety of environmental factors including exercise. Although human beings are expected to grow and develop in a somewhat similar pattern from conception to maturity, each person is an individual, and, therefore, there will be variances in the timing of the growth pattern, and in the amount of growth potential. In fact, children mature at such different rates that chronological age is often a misleading indicator.

The General Growth Pattern

The general growth pattern is characterized by phenomenal growth and development from conception until about two or three years of age. From the age of three until puberty, the growth rate slows dramatically followed by an equally dramatic growth spurt during puberty.

At conception, the newly-formed embryo is microscopic (not visible to the naked eye). Newborns are generally eighteen to twenty-two inches in length, and weigh five to nine pounds. If human beings continued to grow at this prenatal rate, we would be twenty feet tall, and weigh more than the earth by age twenty. By age six, children usually have grown to two-thirds of their adult height. By age twelve, boys have attained 84% of their adult height and girls 93%. The average six year old is three and one-half feet tall, and weighs forty pounds. At age twelve, they are five feet tall, and weigh eighty pounds. Therefore, it takes six years for a child to double his/her weight, and to increase his/her height by one-third.

In the newborn, the head constitutes one-fourth of the total body length, and the legs account for another one-quarter. The remaining fifty percent is, of course, found in the trunk. Human beings would be rather

5

unusual looking creatures if the individual body segments continued to grow at their prenatal rate. This does not occur, because each body part, organ, and system has its own individual pattern and rate of maturity. In the adult, the head accounts for only one-tenth of our height, and the legs fifty percent. Leg growth accounts for two-thirds of the height increase from age one until the onset of puberty.

Childhood (3 - 12 years of age) is characterized by slow but very steady, consistent growth. The middle years of childhood (6 - 12 years of age) are often viewed as non-dramatic in regards to growth, especially when compared to the growth rates of the prenatal, infancy and puberty periods. Yet, the steady growth of this period is critically important as the body tissues mature and develop. Maturity during this period includes the perfection of motor skills which began development during infancy, along with the maturation of the body systems to a point where they can accept the sudden rush to adult status (puberty). During this period, children grow at the rate of two to two and one-half inches per year. Weight gain is usually three to six pounds per year. The child begins to develop a more lean, leggy look, since bone growth tends to be concentrated in the face, arms, and legs. The face becomes more elongated as the lower face and jaw grow to catch up with the head. In general, body features begin to more closely resemble adult proportions. The size and growth rates of boys and girls are comparable until the age of nine or ten as which time girls begin to grow more rapidly.

For both boys and girls, the onset of puberty is signaled by a sudden, short-term decrease in the overall growth rate, and by a sudden increase in the size of the feet. Anyone who has had children will remember this period of time when it seemed impossible to keep the child in an appropriately fitting pair of shoes. Females tend to enter puberty two years in advance of males.

Characteristics of the 6 - 12 Year Old

The brain and nervous system are essentially anatomically mature in most respects by the age of six or seven. At birth, the brain is approximately twenty-five percent of the weight of an adult brain. At six months, it is fifty percent, at two and one-half about seventy-five percent, and ninety percent by age five. Hence, the brain does not grow during the middle years of childhood, but rather develops into a functional system capable of processing information and serving as the command center for the entire organism.

6

The number of muscle cells in the body is complete at birth. Therefore, growth and development of the muscles is a matter of increasing the size, rather than the number, of existing muscle fibers. The muscle cells, thus the muscles themselves, increase in size and strength as they are required to accept a larger workload. Regular physical activity has no apparent effect on stature (overall height), although it is very important in the growth and integrity of muscle tissue. The overall effect is that children progressively increase the ratio of muscle tissue in relation to fat tissue. The rate of change in muscle tissue follows the same growth pattern as that for height. School-aged boys have more muscle tissue than girls, although the difference is not nearly as pronounced as will be noted after the pubescent growth spurt. During the middle childhood years, muscular strength for both boys and girls will, or should, double, yet, muscle tissue at this age is still functionally and anatomically immature.

The growth pattern and rate of the oxygen delivery system (heart, lungs, blood vessels, and blood) follows a growth pattern and rate that is consistent with that of the body as a whole. The heart grows a bit more slowly during these years, and is proportionally smaller than at any other period of life. It is apparent that the components of the oxygen delivery system for children are consistent with those of adults. When physical fitness levels are corrected for body size, research demonstrates that children are capable of obtaining levels of cardiovascular efficiency (aerobic fitness) comparable to adults. Carefully controlled studies show that there are no biochemical or anatomical findings to support the theory that children can be over-loaded to the point of pathological fatigue. This does not mean that a child cannot be involved in an inappropriate exercise regimen. Young males and females are similar in their capacity to develop cardiovascular endurance.

Many professionals are concerned about young athletes who have immature skeletal structures. The formation of bone (ossification) is a complex process, but it can be viewed simply as the replacement of a cartilage frame with hardened bone. The cartilage framework is completed about the eighth week of prenatal development. Shortly thereafter, the ossification process begins, and continues until full skeletal maturity is achieved at about twenty years of age. As mentioned previously, bones mature at different rates. The long bones of the arms, legs, and hands tend to be the bones most susceptible to injury in children. These long bones begin the ossification process in the center of the shaft of the cartilage framework, and also at growth centers near each end. The ends of the bones are also the place where strong muscles attach, rendering this part of the bone more likely to be injured. Damage to any of the growth centers can cause premature termination of bone growth at the site of the injury. Normally, the ossification process proceeds from the growth centers until the entire bone is hardened. There is some evidence that the growing bones and joints of children are more susceptible to certain types of injuries due to the presence of growth cartilage, the muscle/tendon attachments, and the growth process itself. The probability of injury is even greater when the child is growing rapidly.

Implications

Physical activity is essential for normal growth and development although the exact role of regular physical activity in the maturation process has not been clearly established. No studies have been presented which show that even vigorous training and physical stress have any adverse effect on the growth and development of children. Many experts do feel that the amount of physical activity needed for normal growth and development can be attained through free-play activities.

The American Academy of Pediatrics states that sports and exercise have an important positive effect of exercise on a child's stamina and physiological development. It is difficult to separate the effect on growth and development from the normal maturation process itself. However, research does indicate that children who engage in physical training will commonly have wider and stronger bones (bone length is more genetically determined), greater bone density and mineralization, greater muscle tone, better motor skills, and much greater cardiovascular fitness.

If proper techniques of physical conditioning are employed, with workload increases added in a slow, progressive manner, children can engage in exercise and sport without difficulty. Caution and a caring attitude are extremely important when teaching sports skills to children. Attention to proper body mechanics is a must. Remember, most children will appear a little clumsy during late childhood. The legs are growing at a faster rate than other body parts, and the children are not accustomed to maneuvering those fast-growing feet.

8

Heavy resistance weight training programs are not generally recommended for prepubescent children. Programs designed for strength and bulk development should not be used due to the possible negative effect the excessive stress may have on the growth plates located at the ends of the long bones. The desired effect of these strength specialization programs will not likely be realized, because young children lack a sufficient amount of the male sex hormone. If weight training is used, a program of light weights and numerous repetitions will increase muscle tone without placing the bones in jeopardy.

Finally, the American Academy of Pediatrics has concluded that there is no physical reason to separate preadolescent boys and girls by gender in non-collision sports. Programs should take into account the recommendations of such groups.

Chapter III

Psychological Aspects

Daniel Garfinkel and Renee Garfinkel

A marked growth has taken place in organized sports in the seven-to-twelve year old age group over the past thirty years. Along with this growth in sports competition there has been a steady increase in psychological trauma which occurs, not only to the competing youngsters but also to parents and coaches. This chapter focuses on the young athlete as he/she begins his/her team experiences, including the psychological aspects of making or not making the team, coach-player relationships, and how the family learns to relate to the child-athlete.

The Team

There have been several studies performed with youngsters in the 7 - 12 year old age group which deal with the athlete and the "team". Not making the team is extremely threatening to a young child. He/she worries about the loss of friends, how he/she will look in the eyes of peers, etc. Making the team is more important than winning or losing. Once the child is on a team, then it is the team that wins or loses. Research indicates that, with young children, not making a team may be perceived more negatively than such experiences as the death of a grandparent, school suspension, or loss of a job. Other studies indicate that 75% of children surveyed quit a sport because they felt they would not make the team or could not perform up to others' expectations. It is easier for a child to say, "I decided not to try out" than "I tried out and failed". These youngsters sought to drop out because they could not handle the anticipated stress. The coach should know that children should not be traded or released from teams. Youngsters have to feel that they are an important part of the team and equal to their peers.

The Coach

Coaches and managers occupy an important part of the young athlete's life and leave impressions of themselves upon the future life of the youngster. Young athletes often look upon their coaches as God-like people and, in turn, good coaches have a positive influence on the future

10

development of their athletes. Unfortunately, the vast majority of youth sports coaches are untrained volunteers, and problems arise because they have difficulty properly handling the total coaching responsibility.

There has traditionally been concern regarding the effect of organized sports upon the psychological development of the child. Research in this area has shown that coaches gain more respect through knowledge than through personality. Players respect a coach who knows his/her sport and can teach and coach simultaneously. They "see through" the coach who uses jokes and stories, but lacks real know-how in the sport. The knowledge, however, of nontrained, and even some trained coaches tends to be based on their own personal experiences, and is often supported by ill-understood theoretical concepts.

The successful coach can demonstrate positive modes of behavior toward his/her athletes in a variety of ways. For example, the successful coach:

1. gives a positive reaction to a successful performance by one or more players either verbally or nonverbally, i.e., an outstanding player getting a base hit is an expected outcome. However, that player, as well as the unskilled athlete, needs some type of reaction from his/her coach.

2. gives encouragement to a player following a mistake, i.e., the child knows that he/she has not performed as expected. It is up to the coach to remind the child that there is a next time and mistakes can easily be corrected.

3. shows a player who has made a mistake how to do the skill correctly in a specific manner, i.e., the coach who merely yells "that's no way to swing a bat" has taught the athlete nothing. On the other hand, the coach who takes the child aside and repositions his/her hands on the bat or corrects his/her swing has changed a mistake into a learning experience.

4. never makes sarcastic remarks to a player, i.e., a player cannot learn by being ridiculed or belittled either in front of others or privately. Positive reinforcement is the best teacher.

5. never ignores mistakes, i.e., the young athlete knows he/she has made a mistake, and to have it ignored is demeaning. An athlete prefers to be shown what he/she has done incorrectly so that he/she can make an effort to improve his/her performance the next time.

6. always keeps control, i.e., during a traumatizing situation, children tend to become highly involved emotionally, and often look to the coach as a behavior model. It is the stability of the coach which helps the children remain on steady ground.
7. offers encouragement at other times than after a mistake, i.e., when the team is far behind, the coach can help his/her players by acting in a positive manner. Once a coach accepts defeat, the team will follow.
8. is always well-organized, i.e., a coach cannot run an organized team if he/she is not in complete control.
9. has good communication with the players other than at game times, i.e., when a player meets a coach somewhere other than the playing field it raises his/her self-esteem to be recognized, introduced, and acknowledged wherever he/she may be.

Unfortunately, a child who is tagged as a poor athlete may not even get a nod of the head when he/she relates to a coach. It is this child who usually needs more help than the talented athlete. Coaches must be aware of this fact. A favorite story concerns the youngest member of a Little League team. As fate would have it, he was the last batter up in a crucial game that would decide the season champion. The tiny youngster trembled as he approached the plate. He was hoping for the usual walk because of his size. However, the pitcher adjusted to the smaller batter. "Strike one!" A called "strike two!". This time he saw the ball approaching and his dreams of gradeaur sped by. He swung the bat and missed; "strike three" ... end of game. The youngster turned slowly from the batter's box, dragging his bat, with tears streaming down his face. His parents waited apprehensively as the coach took him aside to talk to him. A few moments later, a smiling, happy child came bounding up to his parents saying, "Coach said that was my best swing of the season. If I had connected, it would have been a home run. I can't wait for next year." A smart coach had left the child with a positive attitude and an anticipation of better things to come.

The Parents

Parents should demonstrate to their children that success or failure in a sport does not change their love and respect for the child as a person. Parents should not make the sport experience stressful to the child, and should not be drawing a model for their children from professional sports. "Many are called, but few are chosen", and it is doubtful that a particular child will make it into the big leagues. It is inadvisable to let the child work towards a pro career as his/her only goal in life.

Parents should know to whom they are entrusting their children. They should know the qualifications and personality of the coach. It must be realized that the coach is, in many ways, a surrogate parent and should set forth ideals a child can emulate. On the other hand, parents should refrain from bringing undue pressure on the coach. Volunteer coaches are what makes youth sports "tick". There are areas in the country now where coaching clinics are being held to teach untrained coaches how to work with youngsters. They are taught to improve communications and how to develop a more humane coach/player relationship.

Parents must be made aware of the detrimental effect they may have on the psyche of the child if they are intrusive. They must remember that when the child is on the playing field, the major goal is to have fun and enjoy the experience.

Some Important Concepts to Keep in Mind

1. Coaches, parents, referees, and those working with young athletes must be concerned with not only the physical health, but also the mental health of those children. Community sport programs which improve the youngsters' self-image as well as their physical fitness should be sought out and developed.
2. Focus should be placed on improving communication between players and coaches. This can be done with personal and team meetings. When the young athlete is on the sidelines, the coach and athlete should have individual talks. The coach should relate to the child through positive communication, not ridicule.
3. Intrusive parents should be educated before the season starts so they will refrain from finding fault with the coach or humiliating the child when he/she loses or plays poorly.
4. Parents should let the child athlete be in control of his/her life. The child does not need the added pressure that parents often bring to bear.
5. The child should not be treated as a miniature adult, but as a child.
6. Children should not be made to feel that the sport experience is a measure of their self-worth as a person.
7. Intrinsic rewards, i.e., the joy of playing, should be stressed rather than extrinsic rewards, i.e., trophies, jackets, etc.

Chapter IV

Nutritional Aspects

Gabriel B. Mirkin

Young athletes have basically the same dietary requirements as nonathletes. The main difference is that they may require more food (calories). Provided that they eat a varied diet, they will not benefit from taking nutritional supplements. Bee pollen, wheat germ, protein powders, amino acids, vitamins, and other supplements do not improve health or athletic performance, and may be potentially harmful.

Common Questions

What should the young athlete eat? The primary fuel for muscles during exercise is carbohydrates, such as are found in bread, pasta, fruits, candy, sugar, grains, pancakes and cereals. Therefore, the young athlete should eat a significant amount of carbohydrate-rich foods.

The human body stores carbohydrates (as a complex form of sugar) in the muscles and the liver. How long one can exercise a muscle depends largely upon how much fuel is stored in the exercising muscles. When the muscles run out of their stored carbohydrate supply, they will become fatigued, making it difficult for them to function. Although athletes often attempt to "load up" on carbohydrates prior to competition, it is neither necessary nor desirable that the young athlete manipulate the diet in an attempt to increase carbohydrate stores.

Most well-conditioned athletes do not need to significantly alter their diets. They do so much exercise each day that their muscles are capable of storing more carbohydrates, and will do so with normal carbohydrate intake and precompetition rest. For example, a marathon runner who runs twenty miles per day can maximize muscle carbohydrate storage in only three days by cutting back to five miles per day. No dietary maneuver will increase muscle sugar storage further.

Should the young athlete eat before competition? The athlete should eat breakfast before competition but not to fill the muscles with carbohydrates. Breakfast is eaten in order to provide carbohydrates for liver storage. There is only enough carbohydrate (blood sugar) in the bloodstream to last about three minutes. Muscles and other organs constantly draw sugar for energy from the bloodstream. So, to keep the blood sugar level from falling, the liver constantly releases sugar into the bloodstream. However, there is only enough carbohydrate in the liver to last about twelve hours.

What should the young athlete eat before competition? Virtually anything can be eaten for the pregame meal, provided that it doesn't contain a high amount of sugar. When one eats foods which contain sugar, such as fruits, fruit juices, candy, table sugar and honey, the sugar is rapidly absorbed into the bloodstream. The blood sugar level then rises and when it reaches a certain concentration, the body releases insulin which causes the blood sugar concentration to fall. This can cause the blood sugar level to drop low enough to cause premature fatigue, dizziness and weakness.

Theoretically, the pregame meal should contain very little fat and protein. Fat and protein digest slowly, and may delay the emptying of the stomach, while protein digestion produces organic acids and urea which must be eliminated from the body through the kidneys. Needless to say, the young athlete does not want to have a full bladder during exercise. However, practically, it makes little difference if protein or fatty foods are eaten as long as the stomach is empty at the time the exercise begins. It is suggested that the pregame meal be eaten two to three hours prior to competition.

Finally, it is important that the pregame meal provide adequate fluids to prevent dehydration resulting from strenuous exercise. This is especially critical when the exercise is to be performed in high temperature conditions.

Should the young athlete eat during competition? If an athletic event lasts fewer than two hours, there is probably no need to take in any food during the event. However, if the event takes longer than two hours, extra calories may need to be consumed during exercise. Any sugared drink may be used for this purpose. One need not worry about developing low blood sugar level from taking in sugar during exercise. Muscles will draw the sugar so rapidly from the bloodstream that the blood sugar level will be unlikely to rise enough to elicit an insulin reaction.

Should the young athlete drink during competition? The young athlete should not wait until he/she is thirsty to drink. By that time, a significant water loss will have already occurred. If one is in an event that takes more than an hour to complete, water should be consumed before and every fifteen minutes throughout the event, particularly if the weather is warm.

For events lasting less than three hours, the recommended replacement fluid is simply water. Although there are a large number of "sports drinks" available on the market, the need for such special drinks is controversial, at best. Drinks with a high sugar concentration may be poorly absorbed at rest. However, recent research indicates that most drinks are readily absorbed during exercise. Research also suggests that the temperature of the drink is of little significance, since all fluids between 45 and 80° F appear to be absorbed rapidly into the blood stream.

Should the young athlete eat after competition? After particularly vigorous exercise, the young athlete may feel weak and tired for some time. Several studies have shown that this is, at least in part, due to the delayed replenishment of muscle carbohydrate stores. Therefore, recovery from strenuous exercise may be assisted by eating foods which are rich in carbohydrates.

Other Nutritional Issues

Protein. Athletes do not need to eat large amounts of protein-containing foods such as meat, fish and chicken. Muscles burn fat and carbohydrate for energy. Therefore, there is only a small difference in the amount of protein needed to watch television or sit in the library, and that needed during most exercise.

Taking in extra protein will not enlarge muscles. The single stimulus for making muscles larger is exercise against resistance, such as lifting weights or working out with special strength training machines. This stimulus is so strong that it is possible to enlarge a muscle even when fasting and other muscles are getting smaller.

Furthermore, taking in large amounts of protein can be harmful, particularly in hot weather. As stated earlier, protein digestion results increased kidney function. Therefore, the athlete who consumes extra protein, particularly on a hot day, can become dehydrated and prematurely fatigued during exercise.

Vitamins. Athletes do not need to take extra vitamins. They can get all the vitamins they need from the food they eat. Exercise apparently increases one's requirements for only a very few vitamins, all of which can be found in abundant quantities in food.

Vitamins have specific functions in the body, but are needed in very small amounts. When one takes very large doses of vitamins, the results can be harmful. For example, Vitamin D helps the body absorb and utilize calcium. Large doses (most often associated with taking vitamin supplements) exaggerate this function so that one can absorb so much calcium that kidney stones can result. Niacin helps the liver process carbohydrates. Large doses, however, can cause liver damage and elevated blood sugar levels.

Minerals. Athletes do not need to take extra minerals. As with vitamins, minerals perform very specific functions in the body, and most are needed in very small amounts. One can get all the minerals he/she needs from a balanced diet. For example, years ago, it was believed that the loss of the mineral potassium was a common cause of fatigue in athletes. Potassium is found in almost everything the young athlete eats; fruits, vegetables, meat, fish, chicken, grains, etc. If an athlete develops a potassium deficiency, chances are it is the result, not of exercise, but of illness, vomiting, diarrhea, or the use of diuretics.

Iron. One mineral, iron, may be an exception to the statements above. Iron deficiency, a relatively common problem among American youngsters, may impair athletic performance. Fifty percent of the iron in the body is found in red blood cells. The rest is stored in bone marrow, muscles, liver, and other tissue. One does not become anemic until there is almost no iron outside of the red blood cells. When iron reserves become depleted, the result may be anemia. One out of every five females in this country are iron deficient, although less than one in twenty is frankly anemic.

The best sources of dietary iron are red meat, fish, and chicken. Iron is absorbed very poorly from plant sources, because the type of iron in plants is different from those found in animal sources. There is little concern about getting too much iron from the diet unless the young athlete has a rare hereditary condition called hemochromatosis, which is unlikely.

Vegetarians are more likely to be iron deficient than persons who eat meat. For the nonmeat eater, eggs offer a good source of iron, as do whole grain products which have been fortified with iron. Dried fruits such as raisins, prunes, apricots, and peaches are also excellent sources of iron. The iron content of foods cooked in iron pots may be dramatically increased, although this form of iron is poorly absorbed by the body. One way to improve the body's absorption of iron is to consume foods rich in Vitamin C (citrus fruits and juices, tomatoes, broccoli, etc.) along with iron-rich foods.

Salt. Contrary to popular belief, only on the rarest of occasions will the young athlete require extra salt. The average American takes in ten to twenty times more salt than the body needs on a daily basis.

The young athlete should never take salt tablets on his/her own. As a highly concentrated form of salt, they can irritate the stomach and cause pain. Also, consuming too much salt is far more dangerous than taking in too little. Excessive salt intake has been linked, in some people, with high blood pressure. Furthermore, excessive salt intake can contribute directly to dehydration in the exercising athlete.

On rare instances, a low salt level can contribute to muscle cramps in hot weather. However, the most common cause of such muscle cramps is probably dehydration, combined with a lack of conditioning. If the young athlete develops chronic muscle cramps, consult a physician. A simple blood test can determine if he/she needs more salt.

Eating Sensibly

From the foregoing discussion, it should be evident that there is rarely a need to take dietary supplements. At best, they are a waste of money, and, at worst, they can be harmful. The key to good nutrition for athlete and nonathlete alike is a balanced diet. One of the easiest systems to follow is the four food group plan (high protein foods, milk and dairy products, fruits and vegetables, and grains and cereals) developed by the Department of Agriculture.

Chapter V

Substance Abuse And Eating Disorders

Jerald D. Hawkins

Young athletes, their parents, and their coaches are often as concerned about improving performance as are collegiate and professional athletes. Unfortunately, in their quest for athletic success, young athletes may engage in practices which they (or their parents and/or coaches) believe will improve performance, but in fact may be ineffective at best, or even harmful to the health and well-being of the child. This chapter focuses on two such potentially-dangerous behaviors; substance abuse (including drug abuse) and eating disorders.

Substance Abuse

One of the major health problems in all segments of our culture is substance abuse. Drug-related deaths of college and professional athletes, and suspensions of others for using illegal drugs have shocked us with the knowledge that substance abuse is a serious problem in the athletic community. Even more shocking, however, may be the realization that substance abuse is not confined to collegiate and professional sports. Research indicates that by age 10, one of every three American children will have tried to smoke a cigarette; by age 13, forty percent will have tried wine coolers; and an estimated quarter of a million teenagers currently use anabolic steroids, primarily in an attempt to enhance muscle strength and size. Young athletes, like their adult counterparts, use a variety of substances with the belief that they are ergogenic (work-enhancing, performance-improving — e.g., anabolic steroids, amino acid supplements, etc.), while other substances are used with the belief that they are harmless, and will have little or no adverse effect on health or performance (e.g., tobacco, alcohol, cocaine, etc.). Regardless of the substance or the reason it is used, three critical questions must be addressed: 1) Is it safe, or does it pose a danger to the health of the athlete? 2) Is it illegal? (banned by local, state, or federal law and/or by athletic governing organizations); 3) Will it affect performance (positively or negatively)? Simply stated, research

19

indicates that 1) most substances used by young athletes "ergogenically" and/or "recreationally" are health-threatening, and often life-threatening; 2) many substances used by young athletes are either illegal under law, under regulations of athletic governing organizations, or both; and, 3) even if safe and legal, most substances used by young athletes have been proven ineffective in enhancing performance, and many are detrimental to athletic performance. Therefore, it is imperative that coaches and parents of young athletes play an active role in educating youngsters concerning the potential dangers associated with drug abuse, and be aware of the signs of drug abuse in their young athletes.

The following is a brief discussion of some of the more common substances used by young athletes. A more complete list of common drugs of abuse and their effects is presented in Appendix D.

Tobacco. Tobacco is the number one cause of preventable disease and death in our nation. In spite of this fact, youngsters continue to be fascinated by this substance which is portrayed so glamorously and used so widely in our culture. When professional athletes are seen smoking cigarettes and chewing tobacco, it is not difficult to understand why the young athlete may assume that the use of tobacco is harmless, and will have no adverse effect on his/her performance. The link between cigarette smoking and lung cancer, other cancers, cardiovascular disease, emphysema, and numerous other diseases is clear. The athlete's performance and safety are also jeopardized when he/she chooses to smoke, since smoking decreases the ability to breathe efficiently, reduces the oxygen-carrying capacity of the blood, and accelerates the clotting process, making the athlete more susceptible to blood clots when injured. One of the most common forms of tobacco use among young athletes is chewing or dipping smokeless tobacco. Although traditionally associated with many sports (especially baseball), research shows that the use of smokeless tobacco is not the harmless practice it was once considered to be. Smokeless tobacco (as do cigarettes) contains the strong central nervous system stimulant, nicotine, an addictive drug which is known to contribute to cardiovascular and respiratory disease. Furthermore, smokeless tobacco contains a wide variety of carcinogens (cancer-causing agents), and its use may result in oral and/or throat cancer.

Alcohol. Alcohol is the most commonly abused drug in America, and is often used by athletes (young and old alike) with the belief that it is harmless, and will not adversely affect performance. After all, its consumption is legal (for adults), and current and former sports heroes can be seen starring in beer commercials. However, alcohol is far from being safe and harmless. Among the health risks attributed to alcohol abuse are brain cell damage, increased blood pressure, weakening of the heart muscle, gastric bleeding, peptic ulcers, and liver damage. For the athlete, alcohol poses some special dangers. Not only does alcohol consumption interfere with the development and retention of motor skills (including sports skills), it may impair the liver's ability to synthesize glycogen (the body's stored carbohydrate energy source), interfere with the body's ability to absorb certain essential nutrients, and inhibit the release of antidiuretic hormone, causing excessive fluid loss through urination. In the exercising athlete, this latter effect may produce dangerous dehydration.

Marijuana. In many areas of our country, the use of marijuana is more common among young people than that of alcohol. Unfortunately, this is also true among young athletes. Originally touted as less harmful than other drugs, research now indicates that marijuana use poses dangers once associated only with "harder drugs". Marijuana is an hallucinogenic drug which has been shown to impair short-term memory, interfere with the development of motor skills, and contribute to long-term reproductive problems (especially when used prior to and during adolescence). Further- more, marijuana smoke contains more cancer-causing agents than tobacco, and because it is often inhaled more deeply and held in longer, the risk of lung cancer may be even greater than that associated with cigarette smoking. Finally, the possession and sale of marijuana are illegal, and punishable by fine, imprisonment, or both.

Cocaine. One of the most disturbing trends in today's athletic community is the use of cocaine and/or "crack" (rock cocaine) by athletes. The use of cocaine and "crack" is an addictive and potentially deadly practice, as witnessed by the recent cocaine-related deaths of well-known sports personalities. Also, cocaine's effects on the body can adversely affect an athlete's ability to perform on the playing field. Among these detrimental effects are elevated heart rate, constriction of blood vessels, elevated blood pressure, chronic respiratory inflammation leading to respiratory infections, and possible coronary (heart) artery spasms and sudden heart attack. As with marijuana, cocaine is not only banned by most, if not all, athletic governing organizations, its possession or sale is illegal, and punishable by fine, imprisonment, or both.

Anabolic Steroids. Anabolic steroids are synthetic drugs which function in the body as male hormones. Originally developed for and used by German soldiers in World War II to enhance aggressiveness, they have become popular among athletes who believe they will produce gains in both muscle size and strength. Apparently, in some individuals, and under certain specific circumstances, steroids may produce significant gains in muscle development. However, the risks associated with steroid use far outweigh any possible benefits that may exist.

Research indicates that steroid use may increase one's susceptibility to cardiovascular disease, contribute to liver damage (including tumors), reduce the size and functional ability of a male's testicles, promote degenerative bone and joint disease in adolescents, cause negative personality changes, and inhibit the body's immune system, making the user vulnerable to other disease problems. Experts have recently speculated that the number of cancer deaths among professional athletes will increase dramatically during the coming years as a direct result of steroid use, and its effect on the body's immune system. Anabolic steroids also appear on the banned substance list of all major athletic governing bodies. Finally, recent Federal legislation makes the prescription, sale, distribution, possession, and/or use of anabolic steroids for athletic purposes illegal, and punishable by fine, imprisonment, or both.

Nutritional Supplements. One of the most popular practices among today's athletes is the use of so called "nutritional supplements" in an attempt to improve performance. It has been estimated that more than 85% of the world's athletes use nutritional supplements. The practice of using nutritional supplements to improve athletic performance dates back to ancient times when taking in powdered lion's teeth was believed to enhance courage and drinking blood from the deer was thought to make one run faster. While the supplements used by today's athletes are somewhat more sophisticated, for the most part, they are equally ineffective. With the exception of medically-diagnosed nutritional deficiencies, there is no scientific evidence that an athlete's performance will be improved by taking vitamin supplements, mineral supplements, protein powders, amino acid pills, bee pollen, wheat germ, ginseng, caffeine, or any of the other purported "nutritional ergogenic aids" on the market today. On the contrary, many nutritional supplements are known to actually inhibit physical performance, and many may simply be hazardous to the health of the young athlete.

Recognizing Substance Abuse

Other than prevention, the most effective method of dealing with substance abuse in the young athlete is early detection and prompt intervention. Unlike collegiate and professional sports where drug testing is used, coaches and parents of young athletes must rely on careful observation to detect signs of substance abuse. Some common signs of substance abuse in school-age children are shown in the following.

Signs of Possible Substance Abuse in School-Age Children

1. Change of friends or social groups;
2. Unusual mood swings;
3. Unusual, secretive behavior;
4. Loss of interest in activities;
5. Lack of motivation;
6. Sudden decline in grades;
7. Changes in dress and grooming habits;
8. Marked change in eating habits;
9. Unhealthy appearance, bloodshot eyes;
10. Smell of tobacco, alcohol, marijuana, etc.;
11. Drug-related pictures, drawings, doodling, etc.;
12. Trouble with legal or school authorities;
13. Unusual hostility, irritability, or passivity;
14. Unusual or sudden increase in muscle size/strength;
15. Quick weight gain.

Note: The existence of these signs in combination may be a better indicator of possible substance abuse than the existence of any single sign by itself. Also, these signs may not always be indicative of substance abuse, but may never-the-less, be cause for parental concern.

If a coach suspects that a young athlete is involved in substance abuse, he/she should contact the athlete's parents, and discuss his/her suspicions. A parent who suspects substance abuse should seek medical or other professional guidance. Substance abuse not only jeopardizes the health and well-being of our young athletes, but also threatens to erode the integrity of competitive sports.

Eating Disorders

Among the most disturbing problems facing today's young athletes is the increase in the prevalence of eating disorders. Eating disorders may be defined as pathogenic (health-threatening) behavior patterns characterized by an obsession with thinness, resulting in the loss of inordinate amounts of weight, even to point of death. Research indicates that 90 to 95% of all eating disorders occur in females. It has been estimated that possibly as many as 10 to 15 of every 100 adolescent girls and young females suffer from some form of eating disorder. Young athletes involved in activities which stress body aesthetics (e.g., dance, gymnastics, cheerleading, etc.) and/or maintaining a prescribed weight (e.g., wrestling, some youth football programs, etc.) are at increased risk of developing eating disorders. Therefore, it is imperative that parents and coaches of young athletes understand the serious health threat posed by pathogenic weight control behaviors. The following is a brief discussion of the two most common eating disorders.

Anorexia Nervosa. Anorexia nervosa may be described as an abnormal preoccupation with becoming/being thin, which may begin with simply eating less, and evolve into an addiction, resulting in planned starvation. Although the exact causes of the disease are not clearly defined, the potential consequences are well known. If untreated, anorexia nervosa will result in the progressive deterioration of all major body systems. Approximately 15% of all anorexics die. Furthermore, it has been suggested that fewer than half of those in the latter stages of the disease will show long-term response to treatment. Therefore, early detection and professional treatment are mandatory.

Bulimia. Bulimia (often called bulimia nervosa or bulimarexia) is a disease of addiction in which one binges on calorie-rich foods, then purges (vomits or uses powerful laxatives) in order to lose weight or prevent weight gain. Many, but not all bulimics are also anorexic. In addition to tooth, gum, and esophagus damage resulting from repeated vomiting, the bulimic may experience progressive deterioration of various body systems causing prolonged illness, and even death. As with anorexia nervosa, early detection and professional treatment are critical.

Recognizing Eating Disorders
Early detection and prompt intervention are the keys in successfully managing eating disorders. Parents and coaches of young athletes must be constantly on the look-out for indications of eating disorders. Some common signs of eating disorders in school-age children are shown in the following.

24

Signs of Possible Eating Disorders in School-Age Children

ANOREXIA NERVOSA

1. An exaggerated fear of being overweight or getting fat, even though underweight;
2. Preoccupation with body image and diet;
3. Distorted perception of body image, seeing one's self as fat, even as he/she becomes thinner;
4. Preoccupation with increasing exercise;
5. Skipping meals and/or avoiding eating with others;
6. Wearing bulky clothing in an obvious attempt to hide the contours of the body;
7. Light-headedness and/or fainting without apparent cause;
8. Weight loss during normal growth periods;
9. Mood changes (irritability, depression, etc.).

BULIMIA

1. Signs identified above for anorexia nervosa;
2. Recurrent binge eating without expected weight gain;
3. Reliance on vomiting, laxatives, and/or diuretics for weight loss;
4. Frequent weight fluctuations of more than ten pounds;
5. Frequently excusing one's self immediately after meals to "go to the bathroom", "catch a quick shower", etc., often returning with bloodshot eyes.

Note: The existence of these signs in combination may be a better indicator of possible disordered eating than the existence of any single sign by itself. Also, these signs may not always be indicative of an eating disorder, but may, never-the-less, be cause for parental concern.

If a coach suspects that a young athlete has an eating disorder, he/she should contact the athlete's parents, and discuss his/her suspicions. A parent who suspects that his/her child may have an eating disorder should seek medical or other professional guidance. Furthermore, parents and coaches should exercise extreme caution when making comments, directly or indirectly, about the young athlete's weight or body image, and should never encourage quick weight loss or gain, purging, laxatives, diuretics, sauna suits, fad diets, or any other potentially-dangerous weight manipulation strategy.

Chapter VI

The Young Female Athlete

Mona M. Shangold

Historically, girls have been discouraged from exercising. Too often this attitude has resulted in unhealthy, sedentary, obese adults. Young girls should be encouraged to exercise at an early age. They must learn, as children, that exercise is fun, in order to acquire a regular exercise habit that will last throughout life.

Sensible exercise offers many benefits to girls. Many of the medical problems which are often associated with aging (e.g., thin and brittle bones which break easily, obesity, depression, heart attacks, diabetes, etc.) actually result, at least in part, from inactivity. In order to avoid these medical problems in later life, girls must learn to exercise while young.

Contact Sports

Contact sports are no more dangerous for girls than for boys. A girl's ovaries are located inside her abdomen and are, thus, better protected from possible injury than a boy's testicles, which are vulnerably located in his scrotal sac. Breasts are not particularly vulnerable to injury either. Before they develop, at the time of puberty, they certainly pose no problem. After breasts have enlarged at puberty, most girls find it more comfortable to exercise wearing a bra which provides good support. Many girls with small breasts may prefer to exercise without wearing a bra. Even large breasts pose no medical hazards. Breast injuries are rare, even in contact sports, and most heal very quickly.

Menstrual Problems

Athletic girls often begin to menstruate at a later age than their sedentary friends. This delay poses no medical problems, although some athletic teenagers may experience psychological discomfort from being less sexually developed than their peers. Any girl should be examined by a gynecologist if she has not begun to develop breasts, underarm hair, or pubic hair by the age of 14, or if she has not begun to menstruate by the age of 16. Also, any vaginal bleeding or discharge prior to the age of nine should be evaluated by a gynecologist.

No girl is too young to have a pelvic examination, which should be accompanied by an explanation of exactly what is being done and how it will feel. Any girl is necessarily anxious before having a pelvic examination for the first time. Therefore, special reassurance and support are essential, in order to permit satisfactory examination, to avoid physical discomfort, and to prevent emotional trauma.

An annual pelvic examination is acceptable, although not essential, for any teenagers who have regular monthly periods without problems. "Regular" periods are those which occur every 25 to 35 days, counting from the first day of one period to the first day of the next period. Any girl who bleeds more frequently than every 20 days or less frequently than every 60 days should be examined by a gynecologist. She should also be evaluated by a gynecologist if she stops menstruating altogether, even though this is often associated with heavy exercise. Although it is common for athletes to have irregular periods or stop menstruating altogether, serious problems can also cause these conditions, and it is dangerous to assume that the exercise is the cause without a gynecological examination. Many teenagers stop menstruating when they exercise strenuously or lose weight by dieting, but this menstrual problem must always be evaluated in order to rule out a serious cause. Even if there is no serious cause, some girls may require treatment, in order to prevent a serious result.

Regular exercise is healthful for all girls, both physically and psychologically. None should avoid exercising for fear they will develop menstrual problems, although such problems should be dealt with when they arise.

Chapter VII

Selected Youth Sport Resources

Thomas B. Stevens

There are some three million volunteer coaches in children's and youth sports programs in the United States. The vast majority of these men and women have had little sport-specific training, and little, if any, professional preparation in sport philosophy, sports medicine, sport pedagogy (how to teach), sport physiology, or sport psychology.

Coaching Education

In nations where the government assumes a much stronger role in the development and administration of youth sport, coaches are generally well-trained. Some countries have developed coaching education programs with different levels of training required for positions at various levels of competition. In the United States, for the most part, there are no prerequisites for those who want to coach in children's and youth sports programs. Many experts in this country believe that it is essential that we develop some national guidelines for coaches at all levels, along with an efficient method for disseminating information to prospective coaches of all age groups.

In September, 1989, The First National Coaching Education Conference was held at the United States Olympic Training Center in Colorado Springs. As a result of this conference, a National Coaching Education Task Force was created. The first topic addressed was a mission statement. The group unanimously agreed that the mission of a National Coaching Education Association should be "to enhance the quality of the sport experience by identifying and sharing information to support and improve coaching education". Four levels of coaching education were identified; youth/community, interscholastic, intercollegiate, and national/ international. Coaching education is probably the most neglected aspect of youth sports programs in this country today. Therefore, the education of coaches involved in youth sports programs is the single most effective way to improve children's and youth sports in a country where sport is so important and pervasive.

Resources For Coaches And Parents

Although there is not yet an effective networking system for coaching education in America, there is now an active movement to make this a reality. Today there are several sources of important, reliable, and high-quality materials and information for youth sports coaches and parents, including information on coaching education programs, symposia, and conferences. The following organizations are dedicated to the development of competent and caring youth sports coaches, and are valuable resources for parents, coaches and administrators:

1. Tim Johnson
    National Director
    The American Coaching Effectiveness Program
    Box 5076
    Champaign, IL 61820
    (217) 351-5076 (800) 747-4457 (217) 351-2674 FAX

2. Mike Pfahl
    National Executive Director
    National Youth Sports Coaches Association (NYSCA)
    2611 Okeechobee Road
    West Palm Beach, FL 33409
    (407) 684-1141, (407) 684-2546 FAX

3. Keith Cruickshank
    Amateur Athletic Foundation
    2141 West Adams Boulevard
    Los Angeles, CA 90018
    (213) 730-9600, (213) 730-9637 FAX

4. YMCA, Programs Store
    Box 5077
    Champaign, IL 61825
    (217) 351-5077

5. Paul Vogel
   Positive Approaches to Children's Education (PACE)
   Youth Sports Institute
   213 I.M. Sports Circle
   Michigan State University
   East Lansing, MI 48824
   (517) 353-6689

6. Rick Ball
   Basic Athletic Sports Injury Care (BASIC)
   BASIC Foundation
   9008 N. 14th Drive
   Phoenix, AZ 85021
   (602) 678-0288

As all of these organizations, and others around the country begin to coordinate their efforts, all of our young athletes, both boys and girls, will participate under the guidance of knowledgeable, caring, and philosophically sound coaches.

Chapter VIII

Medical History And Examination

Robert E. Gwyther

To insure the safe participation of the child athlete, most states and many community recreation programs require physical examinations prior to athletic participation. This chapter examines the purposes, nature, and results of the preparticipation physical examination, and discusses common misconceptions which surround the examination process.

Purposes of the Preparticipation Physical Exam

The preparticipation physical exam serves two major purposes. First, it provides the physician with baseline information concerning the athlete's current health status, which can then be used to evaluate subsequent changes in the patient's physical condition, including injuries and illnesses that might occur. Following the preparticipation exam, recommendations are made by the physician concerning the types of activities in which the athlete may safely participate. Second, the physical examination is a valuable tool for providing health counseling or for discovering previously undiagnosed problems, either physical or psychological.

Nature of the Physical Exam

There are many ways in which sports-related physical examinations are conducted, ranging from a personal appointment with one's family physician to mass examinations reminiscent of those physicals performed on military recruits. While the latter serves the purpose of economy and standardization, the personal visit to one's physician who is familiar with the patient is generally recommended. In either case, a standard form should be used for recording the information obtained in the examination.

Results of the Physical Exam

Based upon the physical examination, the physician must make a decision to either grant full approval for athletic participation or choose one of the following four options. First, the doctor may choose to treat an existing condition, and delay his/her decision regarding participation pending the outcome of the treatment. Second, he/she may defer the decision pending examination of the child by a colleague. Third, he/she may approve participation in specific activities. Finally, he/she may disqualify the child from participation.

The following conditions are taken into consideration when making recommendations relative to athletic participation:

1. *Vital Signs.* There are numerous rules of thumb about vital signs which are supposed to trigger suspicion; e.g., unexplained blood pressure over 135/85, or resting pulse rate less than 44 or over 120. In this day of joggers, however, it is well to keep in mind that some athletes have pulse rates in the 40s. Finally, no athlete should participate in vigorous exercise when a fever is present.

2. *Acute Infections.* A variety of acute infections affect most persons, and athletes are no exception. Generally speaking, infections should be treated when possible, and activity levels should be modified so as not to hinder recovery. Special mention of mononucleosis should be made in the case of child athletes because of the accompanying enlarged organs. No athlete should participate in contact sports while the danger of a ruptured spleen is present.

3. *Eyes.* The danger of losing sight in a single, remaining eye must be considered for contact sports. In addition, the history of previous retinal detachment or extreme myopia must be considered in contact sports because of the propensity of those athletes to develop retinal detachment.

4. *Respiratory.* Certain respiratory diseases inevitably present problems for athletes. Asthma, especially exercise-induced asthma, is often a problem, because the athlete can have difficulty maintaining oxygenation of the blood.

5. *Cardiovascular.* Hypertension in children is not common, but needs to be worked up and treated if it is discovered. Essential hypertensives can fully participate in sports, but they should be under treatment and in good control. Heart murmurs in children are commonplace, and most of them are functional. The ones that represent significant lesions of the heart should be identified and worked up appropriately. Hypertrophic cardiomyopathy (pathological enlargement of the heart) is the most worrisome condition, because it can result in sudden death.

32

Exercise is not contraindicated with most lesions causing murmurs, although the child should definitely not be pushed past the limit of tolerance. The presence of sinus bradycardia is not cause for alarm. One tip-off to this condition is that the heart rate slows during inspiration. Other arrhythmias should be diagnosed and treated prior to participation in athletics.

6. *Enlarged Organs.* The presence of an enlarged spleen or liver signals potentially dangerous underlying pathology, and suggests appropriate caution. When these physical findings are present, a diagnosis must be sought. Even if the condition is benign, the risk of rupture must be considered for contact sports.

7. *Hernias.* The presence of ventral or inguinal hernias raises the possibility of incarceration and/or strangulation. Approval for participation in athletic activity can be delayed pending corrective surgery, depending on the nature of the sport under consideration.

8. *Ostomies.* Mechanical damage may be done to certain surgically created structures, especially in contact sports. Thus, the examining physician may want agreement of the surgeon involved prior to giving authorization for participation in contact sports.

9. *Urinary Tract.* The presence of protein in a urine specimen is usually benign, and often disappears on a repeated, first morning specimen. Blood in the urine can be serious, but increasing knowledge about athletic pseudonephritis has lessened concern about hematuria that appears following exercise, and clears with rest.

10. *Nervous System.* A history of being knocked unconscious repeatedly is ominous if the athlete participating in such contact sports as boxing and football, and one which must be carefully evaluated. The history of epilepsy demands attempts at proper control for all athletes, just as for all children. Safeguards should be made for epileptics who swim, or who participate in other dangerous environments.

11. *Hematologic.* The athlete with sickle cell disease (not sickle cell trait) may experience difficulties where hypoxia (shortness of oxygen in the blood) is likely to occur. Athletes with sickle cell trait are generally free from complications during athletic participation.

Misconceptions About the Physical Exam

Unfortunately, as valuable as the preparticipation physical examination is in the child athlete, many misconceptions still exist concerning the process and its benefits. The following are some of the most common misconceptions held by parents and youth sport volunteers:

1. A preparticipation physical exam assures that the athlete has no illness or injury which might post difficulties during athletic participation. FACT: There are many conditions which could interfere with safe athletic participation. The physician has no crystal ball.

2. It is the physician's responsibility to search for some "disqualifying condition". FACT: This idea may have been fostered many years ago by medical textbooks which set forth specific lists of conditions which were believed to be grounds for exclusion from athletic participation. However, today's family physician tries to help children participate in appropriate activities rather than find reasons to totally disqualify them.

3. Once a disqualifying condition is discovered, the child should be kept out of all sports. FACT: Most authorities agree that sports should be categorized according to their level of strenuousness and body contact. Assessment of the risk of participation may then be made within the activity grouping, and recommendations may include approval for participation in some categories while excluding the child from participation in others. The following is an example of classifying sports according to physical demand:

I. Strenuous - Contact

Football
Ice Hockey
Lacrosse (Men)
Rugby
Wrestling
Boxing

II. Strenuous - Limited Contact

Basketball
Field Hockey
Lacrosse (Women)
Soccer
Volleyball
Water Polo

III. Strenuous - Noncontact

Crew
Cross Country
Fencing
Gymnastics
Skiing
Swimming
Tennis
Track and Field

IV. Moderately Strenuous

Badminton
Baseball
Curling
Golf

V. Nonstrenuous

Archery
Bowling
Ping Ping
Riflery

4. A child must have a complete history and physical examination prior to participation in each sport during the year. FACT: If the child participates in more than one sport during the year, it is not necessary to submit him/her to multiple examinations. A single comprehensive examination prior to each year should be sufficient unless injuries or illnesses during that year significantly change the health status of the child. Also, if a child enters an activity which is more strenuous or involves more bodily contact than previous activities, additional examination may be warranted if the initial examination was not comprehensive.

Information in this chapter was obtained from "The History and Medical Examination of the Young Athlete" by Dr. Robert E. Gwyther, The Family Medicine Review, Winter 1982, Volume 1, Number 3. Reproduced with permission.

Chapter IX

Conditioning The Young Athlete

Jerald D. Hawkins

One of the most effective methods of preventing sports-related injuries, as well as improving performance and overall health, is a sound program of physical conditioning. Although rigorous training schedules are usually recommended for the older, more mature sports participant, the young athlete may also benefit from a sensibly-designed and implemented, though less rigorous, exercise program.

Purposes of a Conditioning Program

The major differences between the young sports participant and the older athlete may be found in the extent to which conditioning is necessary to meet the demands of their respective sports, and the ways in which their bodies will respond to physical training. Because of the potentially intense demands of adolescent and adult sports activities, the older athlete must train rigorously if he/she is to perform at a highly-skilled competitive level. While the young athlete may choose to emulate his/her older sports "heroes", it is rarely necessary or desirable for him/her to be subjected to as intense or regimented a training program in order to enjoy participation in youth sports like soccer and football. Furthermore, the young child may not respond in the same manner to some forms of training which, at best, may produce frustration in the child and/or parent, and, at worst, may be harmful to the child. Unfortunately, physical conditioning programs are too often attempts to imitate the methods used by great professional and college coaches rather than creative efforts to meet the specific needs of young children participating in recreational activities. Dr. Jack Wilmore, noted exercise physiologist from the University of Texas, may have stated the issue best when he said, "The conditioning of athletes should involve more innovation and less imitation." This statement was never more true than in the case of the young sports participant.

Physical conditioning should accomplish two distinct purposes in the youth sports program. First, regular exercise should be used to reduce the possibility of injuries resulting from such conditions as premature fatigue and lack of flexibility. Second, youth sports offer the child an excellent opportunity to learn and practice sound exercise habits which will benefit him/her in later years regardless of future sports participation.

Conditioning Guidelines

The oft quoted misconception, "no pain, no gain", has no appropriate place in the youth sports program. The young athlete should learn very early that exercise, while not always pleasant, does not have to be painful to be beneficial. In fact, the more positive one's initial experiences with exercise, the more likely he/she is to incorporate exercise into the daily lifestyle throughout life.

Since injuries are often the result of fatigue, a primary concern of all coaches is the prevention of fatigue in their athletes. Technically, the best method for accomplishing this is through a systematic program of cardiorespiratory (heart and lungs) or aerobic conditioning. Since most young athletes enjoy a more active daily routine than their adult counterparts, it is unlikely that a highly structured conditioning program will be needed in order for the young athlete to be "in shape" to participate. This is especially true in those activities in which a substantial part of each practice session is spent in activities such as skill drills, running plays, and scrimmage games. Even in those circumstances where this is not the case, young children usually engage in other activities such as back yard games and school physical education programs which adequately prepare them for the cardiorespiratory demands of their youth sports activities.

This is not to imply that cardiorespiratory fitness is not important to the health and well-being of the child. Intense conditioning, however, should not be a major part of the youth sport program, since the primary goal of youth sports is not peak performance but, rather, maximum enjoyment.

One of the most common causes of sports-related injuries is the lack of flexibility. Muscles which lack flexibility (the ability to stretch without injury) are more likely to be strained, an injury commonly referred to as a "pulled muscle". Flexibility may be maintained and improved by incorporating stretching exercises into the daily training routine. The most widely recommended method of flexibility training is known as static stretching, a technique by which muscle groups are gradually placed on a stretch and held in that position for 30 to 45 seconds. By contrast, it is not recommended that stretching exercises be done by "jerking" or "bouncing" with the muscles on a stretch, since this tends to tighten the muscle, and may actually promote injury. Some suggested stretching activities are presented in Appendix E.

The young athlete should learn that each exercise session should have three specific segments; warm-up, training activity, and cool-down. These segments should be incorporated into every practice session, especially when a significant level of physical exertion is involved.

The warm-up phase of each session should last 10 to 15 minutes, and should include three specific types of activities. The session should begin with all participants jogging at an easy pace for approximately five minutes to raise the temperature of the muscles, and allow for the gradual adjustment of the cardiovascular system to the impending exercise session. After the job has been completed, the young athletes should stretch for at least five minutes utilizing the types of stretching activities suggested earlier. This will reduce the possibility of muscle strains during the practice or game. The final phase of warm-up should include light forms of physical activity such as general calisthenics and skill-related drills. These will not only further prepare the young athletes for the practice or game activities, but will also serve to promote group spirit and an opportunity for the young players to identify with the activities that they have seen other athletes utilize during pregame warm-up.

As previously stated, for the young athlete, the training activity portion of the exercise session is most often the practice, scrimmage, or game itself. However, the child should learn that this plan should be utilized when any exercise is done. Furthermore, a minimum of 20 to 30 minutes of activity should be included in this phase if cardiorespiratory conditioning is to take place.

The third exercise phase, the cool-down, serves the purpose of allowing the body to gradually return to its pre-exercise state, rather than stopping the activity abruptly. This segment of the workout should last approximately 5 to 10 minutes, and should include light, fun activities such as walking while tossing a ball or frizbee, shooting free throws, or simply repeating the stretching activities to relax muscles which may have become tight during the practice or game.

Common Questions

The following are some questions which are commonly asked relative to conditioning and the young athlete:

1. *What about weight training for the young athlete?* Weight training is one of the most effective methods known for developing stronger and larger muscles. However, the development of both muscle strength and muscles size depend to a large extent upon the existence of a significant amount of certain hormones in the body. These hormones are generally not present in significant amounts until the young athlete enters puberty. Therefore, most authorities agree that weight training prior to thirteen or fourteen years of age (or until signs of puberty appear) is not generally recommended since the desired results are less likely to be realized, often leading to disappointment and frustration in the athlete. Also, the young athlete is still in the midst of his/her developmental years, and the bones and joints are subject to injury from extreme stress or trauma. This is another reason that many experts discourage the use of heavy weights in an attempt to improve the musculature of the preadolescent athlete.

2. *Will athletic participation cause a young girl to develop a masculine appearance?* There is no reason to be concerned that young female athletes will develop "ugly muscles" or other "masculine" traits. As stated earlier, the development of large muscles is largely dependent upon male hormone influence in the body along with the results of heavy weight training. Most females have only small amounts of these hormones in their bodies, so that even heavy training will be unlikely to produce large, bulky muscles, but rather, healthy, attractive ones.

3. *Is heavy cardiorespiratory training harmful to young athletes?* While the demands of youth sports programs should not, and usually do not require high levels of cardiorespiratory efficiency, many young people choose to engage in activities such as distance running and swimming. Scientific evidence suggests that a child who is healthy will probably respond positively to rather heavy exercise demands such as those involved in running distances of five miles or more. It is, however, important to note that any such training program should be initiated with professional instruction and supervision, and only as long as it is consistent with the child's interests and desires.

4. *Are there unsafe conditioning activities for young athletes?* There are several activities which are potentially unsafe for anyone, and should be avoided when working with young athletes. Among the most common "dangerous" exercises are those which involve "deep knee bends", since placing the knees under stress in an extremely flexed position may promote "looseness" of the joint, a potential source of future injury. Examples of this type of exercise are deep knee bends, toe touch/rocking chair exercises, and duck walks. A second group of activities known to be potentially harmful are those which place stress on the lower back. The two most common offenders are straight-leg sit-ups and leg lifts. However, they should be done with the knees bent and feet flat on the floor or ground. This removes the stress which is placed on the lower back when sit-ups are done with the legs extended. Likewise, lying on the back with the legs straight, and then attempting to lift the feet off the floor or ground also produces adverse stress on the lower back. For this reason, these exercises should be eliminated from the conditioning program.

The youth sport participant (as should any person) should be in good physical condition in order that he/she might enjoy optimal health. However, strenuous physical training should not be a major part of the youth sports program, and when physical training is involved, it should be undertaken in a reasonable and prudent manner.

Chapter X

General Injury Management

Stanley L. Grosshandler

A major concern for any youth sport program should be the prevention of injuries to the participants. It is obvious, however, that even the most carefully designed injury prevention plans will not eliminate sports-related injuries entirely. In fact, sports medicine professionals agree that injuries will always be associated with competitive sports. Therefore, every person who works with young athletes should recognize his/her responsibility for learning proper techniques for caring for injuries when they do occur.

Injury Care Responsibilities

Although every youth sport worker should have a basic knowledge of injury care, each team should have one person designated as having primary responsibility for injury care during practices and games. This person should assume the following general responsibilities:
1. Become trained and certified in basic first aid and cardiopulmonary resuscitation (CPR).
2. Become familiar with the medical history of each player, including past injuries, chronic conditions, allergies, etc.
3. Maintain an adequately stocked athletic first aid kit (see Appendix B).
4. Evaluate and give immediate care for injuries.
5. Transport or arrange for transportation of injured players to a medical facility when such a move is deemed necessary.
6. Notify parents of injured players.
7. Determine whether an injured player may safely return to activity (with the assistance of the physician or parents when appropriate).
8. Maintain records concerning injuries and care provided.

On-the-Field Evaluation

When a player is injured in a game or practice situation, only the person responsible for injury should go onto the field or court. Several people rushing to the injury scene may result in needless confusion and cause unnecessary concern to the injured player and the player's parents. The primary concern at this point is to determine if the injury is such that the player should not be moved. In such cases (e.g., head and/or neck injuries, obvious fracture, etc.), play should be suspended until medical assistance (a physician, emergency medical services, etc.) can be obtained. Fortunately, most injuries are not life-threatening, and once a cursory evaluation of the injury has been completed, the player may be moved to the sideline for further evaluation. Based upon the results of the evaluation as detailed in the following chapters of this book, the player may then be:

1. allowed to remain in the activity if no further danger from the current injury exists.
2. allowed to return to the activity following the completion of further evaluation and/or care, if such action removes the probability of further danger from the current injury.
3. withheld from further activity pending evaluation of the injury and clearance for return by a physician.
4. transported to a medical facility for further evaluation and care.

On-the-Field Injury Care

The following chapters in this book are dedicated primarily to the recognition and care of specific injuries. However, some general guidelines for injury care should be understood before detailed techniques are presented.

Orthopedic Injuries. Orthopedic injuries (those involving bones, muscles, tendons, ligaments, and joints) are most often of the contusion (bruise), sprain, and strain types, although fractures and dislocations may occur. The standard recommended procedure for caring for such injuries may be easily remembered by recalling the word **"R-I-C-E-S"**.

R   **Rest** – Most injuries respond favorably to rest.
I   **Ice** – Most orthopedic injuries tend to swell. Since swelling delays the healing process, ice should be used to slow swelling and provide temporary pain relief. Although common practice, heat should never be applied to a recent orthopedic injury since it will promote swelling and retard healing.
C   **Compression** – Most orthopedic injuries should be wrapped with an elastic wrap to provide pressure and retard swelling.
E   **Elevation** – Elevating (raising) an injured body part by resting it on a pillow or other elevated surface will also help reduce the possibility of swelling.
S   **Support** – Many orthopedic injuries (especially suspected fractures and dislocations) should be supported with a splint or sling to prevent further injury.

In most cases, the **R-I-C-E-S** regimen should be used for the first 24 to 48 hours following the injury, or until active swelling has been controlled. If swelling persists when this procedure is discontinued, the **R-I-C-E-S** plan should be continued.

Exposed Wounds. Among the most common of all sports-related injuries are abrasions (scrapes), lacerations (cuts), and puncture wounds. The initial concern with lacerations is the control of bleeding. The most effective method of controlling bleeding is the application of pressure directly over the wound using a sterile gauze pad. The primary concern with abrasions and puncture wounds, and the second area of concern in lacerations is the prevention of infection. Since the threat of infection often poses a more serious danger than the original wound itself, care should be taken to clean all open wounds thoroughly with antiseptic soap and water. Alcohol or hydrogen peroxide may then be used to further cleanse and disinfect the wound. All open wounds should be bandaged using sterile bandage materials. During the healing process, the player may find that a foam pad worn over the bandage will help protect the wound from further damage.

Two special notes should be considered. First, if there is any question about whether a laceration should have stitches, the player should be referred to a physician for evaluation as quickly as is feasible; certainly within the first 12 hours following the injury. Second, because puncture wounds tend to be deep with a small external opening, there exists a chance of a foreign body being embedded in the wound. Therefore, it is recommended that all puncture wounds be referred to a physician for evaluation and care.

Heat Illness. In those areas of the country where temperature and humidity tend to become very high (90°+ and 80% respectively), heat illness is a threat to the well-being of the young athlete. The most common form of heat illness is muscle cramps, usually occurring in the calves. These may be effectively reduced by applying a steady, firm grasp to the cramping muscle or by gently kneading the muscle. Once the cramp has subsided, gentle stretching may be used. Also, since cramps are often heat-related, the athlete should be given fluids (water, electrolyte drink, etc.) to replace lost body fluids.

Heat exhaustion is a more serious form of heat illness in which the body temperature may become quite high. The player will continue to perspire,

43

and may complain of headache, dizziness, nausea, and/or may vomit. Any player experiencing such symptoms on a hot day should be rapidly cooled by removing excess clothing, fanning, and/or sponging with cool, water-soaked towels.

Heat stroke is the most serious form of heat illness, and may be potentially fatal. Therefore, its symptoms must be quickly recognized, and appropriate actions taken. The player suffering from heat stroke will usually have a temperature of 104° or more, and will have hot, dry skin. The player may develop seizures, and lapse into a coma. He/she must be rapidly cooled by removing all unnecessary clothing, fanning with towels or similar items, and/or sponging with cold water towels.

Victims of both heat exhaustion and heat stroke should be taken immediately to a medical facility for treatment, and should be given fluids, usually by the intravenous route. Also, while it is true that heat illness is often accompanied by a loss of sodium from the body, salt tablets should never be used in the prevention or care of heat illness unless specifically ordered by a physician.

Cardiopulmonary Resuscitation. Cardiopulmonary resuscitation (CPR) is a technique used for restoring blood circulation and/or breathing to a person whose heart and/or lungs have ceased to function. While sports-related injuries rarely result in cardiac and/or pulmonary failure, every person who works with young athletes should learn CPR techniques through classes offered by the American Heart Association and the American Red Cross.

Diseases. Many children are denied the opportunity to participate in sports because of the existence of a disease. While it is recommended that a child not exercise vigorously when he/she is ill, especially if a fever is involved, many chronic diseases such as diabetes and some types of asthma may respond quite favorably to exercise. Many other conditions may also allow for normal sports participation without undue risk to the child. There have been numerous successful professional athletes who have had diabetes, asthma, sickle cell trait, convulsive disorders, and many other such diseases. The family physician should be consulted prior to making a decision about sports participation based upon the existence of disease.

Common Injuries. Some of the more common types of sports-related injuries are not easily classified under the specific topical headings found in this and other sports medicine publications. Therefore, a brief discussion of them is appropriate at this time.

Due to any one of a number of causes, including excitement, a player may simply faint. When a player faints, he/she should be allowed to remain lying down with the feet slightly elevated to increase blood flow to the heart and brain. If breathing and pulse are normal, the player should regain consciousness spontaneously in a matter of seconds or minutes. The process should not be hastened by shaking or slapping the child, or pouring water on the face. Simply calling the child's name while remaining calm will usually do the trick. If consciousness does not return, medical assistance should be sought.

One of the most common injuries, especially in contact sports, is the nose bleed. Nose bleeds may result from a blow to the nose, in which case the possibility of nasal fracture must be considered, or the nose may simply begin to bleed without apparent cause. In either case, the player should be placed in a semi-reclined position, and pressure applied to the side of the nose to close the nostril. In most cases, bleeding will cease within five minutes. If bleeding persists and cannot be controlled, the player should be taken to a medical facility.

"Red Flag" Emergencies. The following conditions should be considered "red flag" emergencies, and should be referred immediately to professional medical personnel for evaluation and care:
1. Absence of breathing (Establish an open airway and initiate rescue breathing or CPR, as needed);
2. Absence of pulse (Initiate CPR);
3. Unconsciousness with inability to arouse;
4. Convulsions;
5. Excessive bleeding;
6. Severe head and/or neck pain, especially with dizziness, nausea, and/or vomiting;
7. Difficulty breathing or significant wheezing;
8. Heat exhaustion and heat stroke.

Finally, the manner in which a coach or parent responds to an injury may have a significant effect on the way in which the injured player reacts. Parents and coaches should remain calm when dealing with an injured player to avoid creating needless emotion and apprehension. Even if a serious injury is suspected, calm reassurance and quick action will prove the most effective way to help the injured child.

Chapter XI

Infectious Diseases

Mark A. Bartz

Exercise and sports participation are activities which contribute to a healthy and enjoyable life. Throughout our lives, we encounter infectious diseases. Many of these diseases can be passed to others, and will not discriminate between the young athlete, his/her family, coach, or teammates. This chapter will examine some common infectious diseases, and preventive measures which may be utilized by parents and coaches. The information presented in this chapter is not intended to include all infectious diseases which involve young athletes, but those about which parents and coaches most often have questions.

Respiratory Tract Infections

Infections of the respiratory tract can involve the mouth, throat, nose, ears, sinuses, and lungs. The ability to maintain an open airway is mandatory to sustain life. When participating in sports, the athlete needs more oxygen to function, and many respiratory tract infections will impair the ability to breathe. Any young athlete suffering from any of the following symptoms should be seen by a physician:

1. Temperature greater than 101° F;
2. Difficulty breathing;
3. Persistent cough;
4. Green or yellow nasal congestion;
5. Unexplained facial pain, chest pain, or throat pain.

A common cold will usually resolve in a few days with rest and treatment for the worst symptoms such as cough, headache, and congestion. If a child is too sick to attend school, he/she is too sick to participate in athletics. Children with high temperatures (101°+F) should not resume sports participation until at least 24 hours have passed without any further temperature elevation.

Infections of the ear or sinuses may cause trouble with balance and; or produce pain without any increase in temperature. This child should be watched carefully prior to allowing his/her return to participation. In lung infections, such as bronchitis and pneumonia, as a child breathes faster and harder, he/she will develop a bad cough, and the physician should determine when a return to sports participation is appropriate.

Failure to properly treat common respiratory infections in the early stages of the illness may result in lost school and sports participation days, and can endanger the overall health of the child.

Viral Infections

Rubeola (Red Measles). Rubella has become more common in the last five to ten years. It is a viral infection which may attack at any age, but is most common among teenagers and young adults. Measles, like many other viruses, is spread by droplet infection. Therefore, if someone coughs, the spray that is projected from the nose and mouth contains the infectious virus.

Persons infected with measles will have fever, runny nose, and a severe cough, and their temperature can get as high as 104-105°. The measles rash will appear as red spots, usually beginning on the neck and face, and spreading to the body, arms and legs. The child will be contagious to those not vaccinated, and should be given bed rest, and isolated from the general public until recovery. The issue of proper measles vaccination should be discussed with a physician in order to prevent measles infection in young children and teenagers.

Rubella (German or Three-day Measles). Rubella is also a viral illness which may be spread by droplet infection, and is more common among teenagers and young adults. The Rubella rash is similar to that of Rubeola, beginning on the neck and face, and spreading to the rest of the body. Unlike Rubeola, however, temperatures generally do not exceed 101° F, and the rash usually disappears by the third day.

Proper vaccination is very important for individual health, and to protect the unborn babies of pregnant females, since there are serious birth defects associated with Rubella infection during pregnancy.

Varicella (Chicken Pox). Varicella is another extremely contagious viral illness which may be spread by droplet infection and/or direct contact with the rash. The initial lesions of chicken pox will be small, clear blister-like bumps. They generally appear on the trunk of the body first, then spread to the head and on to the arms and legs. New lesions will continue to appear for several days. An infected person will be contagious from 24 hours before the rash appears until all areas of the rash are crusted over; usually a total of seven to eight days. Chicken pox can be mild, or can cause fever of 103-105° F, and have secondary complications. A person should be at home until no longer contagious, and should return to school and athletic participation only after being released by a physician.

Infectious Mononucleosis. Infectious mononucleosis (mono) is caused by the Epstein-Barr virus, and can cause fatigue, fever, sore throat, and swollen lymph glands. Most commonly it infects teenagers and young adults, but can also infect other age groups. The virus is spread by exchange of saliva. From the time of contact with the virus until the actual disease begins (incubation period) may be thirty to fifty days. Many people infected with mono feel as though they simply have a mild case of flu, while others may have high fever (101-103° F), feel extremely ill, and take weeks to recover.

Approximately fifty percent of people with infectious mononucleosis will have enlargement of the spleen, an organ located in the upper portion of the abdomen. Those with splenic enlargement should refrain from athletic activity, since a blow to the abdomen can result in rupture of the enlarged spleen and internal bleeding. If the mono patient experiences sudden abdominal pain, he/she should be taken immediately to a physician. A medical release should be received from a physician prior to returning to athletic participation.

As a rule of thumb, if a child has a sore throat, with or without fever, which has not improved within 48 hours of treatment with an antibiotic, a physician should be contacted, and consideration given to testing for infectious mononucleosis.

Acquired Immunodeficiency Syndrome (AIDS). AIDS is a disease caused by the human immunodeficiency virus (HIV). Contrary to popular belief, this virus is spread only by direct contact with bodily fluids; most commonly blood, though other fluids may also transmit the virus. At the time of its origin in this country in the early 1980s, the disease was believed to be unique to IV drug abusers who shared needles, homosexuals, people of Haitian origin, and those exposed to infected blood products. It is now known, however, that anyone can become infected with the HIV virus, including heterosexuals in all age groups.

Each day the body's immune system fights disease, or repairs and replaces worn out and defective parts within the body. A person can carry the HIV virus, yet not develop the Acquired Immunodeficiency Syndrome (AIDS). When an HIV carrier becomes an AIDS sufferer, the immune system has been damaged by the virus to the point where cancers and/or uncommon infections occur. AIDS at this point in time is a terminal disease. Questions about AIDS should be discussed with a physician.

People who have the HIV virus in their bodily fluids are infectious to others, but often have not developed the illness, and may not be known to be carrying the virus. Although the HIV virus is communicable through the direct exchange of body fluids, there appears little, if any, chance of HIV infection during sports participation. However, it is recommended that exposure to blood on the playing field (or elsewhere) be minimized through the use of disposable gloves and the secure bandaging of all injuries. Also, blood on playing surfaces, equipment, etc. should be promptly cleaned up using a 50/50 bleach and water solution. Disposable gloves should be worn during blood clean-up. Additional information concerning the prevention of HIV infection may be obtained by contacting the Centers For Disease Control's toll free National AIDS Hotline at 1(800)342-AIDS.

Other Infectious Diseases

Tick-borne Disease (Rocky Mountain Spotted Fever and Lyme Disease). Tick-borne diseases are caused by infection from a tick bite. Rocky Mountain Spotted Fever (RMSF) is caused by the wood or dog tick. Approximately one to eight days after the tick bite, the infected person may develop headache, fever, muscle aches, fatigue, and a rash. The rash usually appears as small red spots, starting on the ankle and wrist areas, and spreading to the rest of the body. Even if there is no recollection or evidence of a tick bite, a child with these symptoms should be taken to a physician for evaluation and care. If not treated in the early stages, RMSF can be a life-threatening illness.

Lyme Disease is spread by the deer tick, a very small tick which is often not seen by those who are bitten. The Lyme Disease rash appears as a red area at the site of the bite. This rash slowly enlarges over a two to four week period, with redness on the edge of the rash, and clearing in the middle. It will generally disappear over time. If such a rash appears, or if one works or plays in tick-prone areas, and experiences new joint aches, headaches, or fatigue, a physician should be consulted.

In the spring, summer, and fall, children and pets who play in wooded areas or high grass should be carefully inspected for ticks when they return home. This includes young athletes who venture into woods or high grass to retrieve a ball, or routinely walk to and from the playing field through grassy or wooded areas. Any tick should be removed wearing disposable gloves, and using tweezers. The date the tick is discovered should be marked on a calendar to provide the physician helpful information.

Rabies. In many parts of the country, the number of rabid animals being reported is increasing. Rabies is a disease which is transmitted in the saliva of an infected animal. If a person bitten by a rabid animal is not treated, and develops rabies, the result is virtually 100% fatal. Anyone bitten by a wild animal (including bats) should be seen by a physician immediately. When bitten by a domestic animal (dogs, cats, etc.), if the animal has not been properly vaccinated, it should be watched for ten days, and the bite reported to local authorities and a physician. If the animal is captured or killed, the head of the animal should not be damaged, as the brain must be examined for the presence of rabies infection. Any animal bite should be discussed with a physician the same day of the bite, to determine if there is a need for rabies vaccination.

Chapter XII

Skin Problems

John H. Hall

The skin is the external organ of the body. It regulates heat and cold, protects from trauma, provides a barrier to the invasion of bacteria, viruses, and fungi, and performs several other lesser functions.

Contagious Disease

Athlete's Foot (Tinea Pedis). There are several types of athlete's foot. It may be dry, scaly, or very inflamed with oozing and crusting. Sometimes actual blisters are present. It is not as contagious as most people think, but when contagion occurs, it is frequently in a locker room setting or where there is an exchange of foot wear between two people. Simple cases do not involve painful damage to the skin or secondary infection, and can frequently be cured by topical preparations available in any drugstore (e.g., clotrimazole as a cream, or miconzaol as a spray).

Jock Itch (Tinea Cruris). This is usually red and tender, often with scaling and frequently involves both sides of the groin. It, too, can be spread by exchange of athletic supporters or underwear, or transferred from athlete's foot to the groin. Cleanliness is rarely the problem, and treatment should follow as for athlete's foot above. Care should be taken to select a medication which, as stated on the label, is appropriately intended for use on "jock itch" or Tinea Cruris. As with any fungus infection, if severe enough, a prescription medication may be required.

Warts. All warts are caused by the same basic virus, although there may be different types of this virus. Warts are contagious, and frequently more so than the other conditions discussed in this chapter. Their spread often occurs within the same family. Rarely should athletic activity need to be curtailed because of their presence, but usually it is advisable to have them treated. This may usually be postponed until the end of the athlete's current season. The plantar wart is nothing more than a wart growing on the plantar aspect or sole of the foot. While wart medications are available over the counter, these frequently fail or result in secondary infection. Therefore, it is often necessary to have warts treated by a skin specialist (dermatologist).

51

Molluscum Contagiosum. This condition is characterized by pink, dome-shaped bumps which are smaller than a pea, and often multiple in appearance. This is another virus similar to the wart virus, as it involves the skin, and can spread on the same person or to other people. These are simple to remove, but usually require treatment by a dermatologist.

Staph Infection. This term refers to a multitude of simple skin infections, including styes, boils, impetigo, and paronychia (infection around the nail), and may occur any place on the body. These conditions are contagious, and usually require antibiotic therapy. However, the use of antiseptic cleanser by the individual and/or his/her teammates may be useful in reducing contagion. Temporary (and occasionally, curative) treatment involves applying an antibiotic ointment (generic triple antibiotic ointments are available at most drugstores), and covering with a band-aid. Infection resulting in a red streak extending several inches on the arm or leg usually requires prompt prescription or injectable antibiotic therapy, and should, therefore, be referred to a physician.

Herpes (Cold sores, fever blisters, etc.). Although there is a wide variety of herpes conditions, "venereal" or genital herpes is often the most publicized. Genital herpes is contagious. Substantial concern has been created by the media regarding this viral infection, much of which is unwarranted. It should be emphasized that herpes is only sometimes venereal in origin, and that most herpes is not venereal at all. Rarely does it cause any problems other than a local tenderness of the lesions for a limited period of time. Prescription treatments are available; if herpes becomes a problem, medical attention should be sought. Herpes infection of the eye is rare, but curable if treated promptly. However, delay could result in loss of sight. Those involved in sports medicine should be especially aware of herpes virus spreading in the direct contact sports, especially wrestling, where the virus can be inoculated onto an extensive area such as the back from an infected wrestling mat. Traditionally, this has been called "herpes gladiatorium" or herpes of the gladiator. Because of the contagious nature of herpes, an athlete with active lesions should be excluded from participation in contact activities for five to seven days, or until the lesions have healed over.

Scabies. This is a rather contagious chigger-sized mite that produces multiple small, severely itchy bumps. Though frequently found in the area of underclothing, this condition can occur most any place on the body. Scabies should be treated by prescription medication, and any close contacts of the athlete should also be treated.

Lice (Head lice, crab lice, body lice – pediulosis). These, too, are contagious, usually through contact or exchange of clothing items of the involved area. It should be noted that head lice do not transfer to the groin or pubic area, and vice-versa. These conditions may be treated by prescription medication quite effectively, and, after treatment, present no problem of contagion.

Trauma

Blister. A blister is an acute friction trauma causing serum to separate the damaged skin from its dermal base. Treatment usually involves taping a soft pad over the rubbed area. Because of the danger of infection, blisters should be kept intact whenever possible.

Callus. This is a localized thickening of the skin, usually on the plantar aspect of the foot. Frequently caused by poor-fitting shoes, calluses often develop from continued pressure on the same spot regardless of footwear. The condition is usually controlled by paring the callus to a flat and unthickened state with a callus file or emery board. Caution should be used in recommending harsh acid plasters in its treatment. While protection with any soft padding should give relief, prevention is the key to effectively managing calluses.

Soft Corn. A soft corn is a tender, soft callus often found between the fourth and fifth toes. Deep infection can result. Therefore, careful paring and antibiotic ointment may prevent this. Cotton between the toes will reduce the occurrence.

Human Bite. Human bites should be cleansed with hydrogen peroxide (commercially-available 3% strength is adequate). If the wound is deep, consultation with a physician is indicated as these can become dangerously infected.

Sunburn. The best treatment for sunburn is prevention. Fair complexioned athletes should be advised to use a sun lotion available in any drug store. Athletes who do not tan easily, even with prolonged and repeated sun exposure, should use a higher strength sun screen (SPF 20 to 50). Athletes whose hand agility is important should use nongreasy, alcohol-based sun lotions. Aspirin helps reduce the tenderness and redness of sunburn, but usually requires three or four regular adult-sized tablets repeated every three to four hours, and such treatment should not be

53

prolonged. Benzocaine-containing creams and sprays should not be used. It should be noted that sunburn can definitely be treated with substantial improvement and reduction of pain and symptoms. This is frequently done by a dermatologist, and occasionally by other physicians.

Miscellaneous

There are numerous other conditions which may develop which are peculiar to an individual sport or trauma, such as surfer's nodules and black dot toe. Usually, sports physicians, trainers, and coaches become quite familiar with some of these minor disabilities that develop on athletes under their supervision and care.

Whirlpool baths can be the source of spread in many of the contagious conditions discussed in this chapter. Proper levels of antiseptic chemicals will minimize this threat.

Occasionally, an athlete develops a skin inflammation from gear or equipment called allergic contact dermatitis. This condition will persist and worsen until the contactant is removed, changed, or prevented from remaining in contact with the skin. Allergy to tennis shoes, metals, shoulder pads, or gloves can occur.

The common condition of acne can be aggravated substantially by occlusive warm up wear or multiple layers of clothing, especially on the back. The development of inflamed cystic acne frequently requires specialized care of a dermatologist. Similarly, acne can be aggravated under a helmet or a chin strap, and under similar situations where perspiration and friction may aggravate the condition.

Finally, athletes with "eczema" or atopic dermatitis or a history of this in childhood are subject to rapid cooling of the extremities in temperatures that do not cause excessive heat loss in the average person. These athletes frequently note a decreased agility when participating in cooler weather. Most of this loss of agility can be prevented by encouraging the warming of the hands in gloves, and using hand warmers or hot water bottles when not in active participation.

Chapter XIII

Facial Injuries

L.L. Patseavouras

Injuries to the face alone seldom result in death. However, restoration of facial appearance and function requires attention since man's face is his single most distinquishing physical characteristic. Athletic accidents are the second most common cause of facial injuries.

Types of Injuries

Injuries to face may be divided into two basic groups; injuries to the soft tissue, and injuries to the bone. The eye is a specialized organ, injury to should be considered as associated trauma, and will be discussed in detail in Chapter 15.

Soft tissue wounds resulting from athletics are quite different from those seen following automobile accidents. The most common are lacerations, abrasions, hematomas, and puncture wounds. Lacerations of the face may be of a simple, tearing type. Forces exerted over the external ear, as seen in wrestling or boxing, may result in hematoma (a collection of blood) formation. If not treated properly, these hematomas can eventually result in cauliflower ears, characteristically seen in wrestlers and boxers. These injuries may be minimized by the use of properly fitted protective headgear. In soft tissue injury, immediate treatment consists of application of pressure over the injury if bleeding is present. Otherwise, covering the wound with a sterile bandage until definitive treatment can be carried out is generally recommended.

Injuries to facial bones can best be considered by dividing the face into thirds. The upper third consists of the frontal bone, and extends to the superior orbital wall (level of the eyebrows). The frontal sinus and supraorbital ridge are the most common fractures in this area.

The middle third of the face contains the greatest concentration of facial bone structures; the orbit, the nose, the palate, and the maxillary sinuses. Fractures of the middle third of the face are the most difficult to diagnose and treat. The most prominent facial bones would be expected to be the most commonly injured, and this has proven statistically to be true. Nasal bones are most commonly fractured. The zygoma/malar (cheekbone) fracture is the next most frequent type of fracture, with fractures of the orbital rims and orbital floors commonly occurring in association. The zygomatic arch can be fractured independently. Maxillary teeth and the alveolar process are included in the middle third of the face.

The lower third of the face consists only of the mandible (lower jaw bone) and the teeth supported by it. These offer numerous, but generally predictable sites for fractures.

Evaluation of Facial Injury

After control of the patient's general condition, the facial injury can be evaluated and treated. Evaluation may be accomplished by the following three techniques:

Observation. Observation of facial injury begins with the surface for indications of soft tissue injury. Evaluation of facial symmetry should be next, noting any imbalance which could be due to injury.

Palpation. Palpation (feeling) of bony prominences of the face bilaterally is especially helpful, especially in fractures of the cheekbone. Tenderness is a clue to the site of a facial bone fracture, but seldom is discomfort intense.

X-ray Examination. Gross facial bone fractures can usually be diagnosed without x-ray confirmation, and some grossly displaced facial bone fractures will not visualize well on x-ray. Yet, x-ray studies play a definite part in the evaluation of facial injuries.

As attention is focused on each of these areas, certain observations should be noted:

1. Supraorbital and lateral orbital rims (above and alongside the eye)
   a. Bony depression or deformity;
   b. Tenderness;
   c. Eyebrow irregularity;
   d. Eye prominence or smaller appearing;
   e. Ecchymosis (sign of hemorrhaging);

f. Double vision;

g. Numbness of forehead.

2. Infraorbital rims (below the eye)
    a. Depression or deformity;
    b. Tenderness;
    c. Bruising;
    d. Double vision;
    e. Numbness in adjacent bones.

3. Malar Eminences (cheekbone)
    a. Comparison of heights;
    b. Bruising;
    c. Deformity.

4. Zygomatic Arches (below the temple and above the cheek)
    a. Depression or deformity;
    b. Ecchymosis;
    c. Tenderness;
    d. Limitation of jaw movement.

5. Nasal Bones
    a. Depression or deformity;
    b. Ecchymosis;
    c. Nose bleed;
    d. Tenderness.

6. Maxilla (upper jaw)
    a. Dental malocclusion (teeth do not meet properly when the mouth is closed);
    b. Bruising;
    c. Movement of the maxilla;
    d. Missing or damaged teeth;
    e. Tear of cheek mucosa or palate.

7. Mandible (lower jaw)
    a. Tenderness and pain;
    b. Asymmetry of mandibular contour;
    c. Asymmetry of dental arch;
    d. Dental malocclusion;
    e. Limitation of movement;
    f. Misplaced or damaged teeth;
    g. Numbness of teeth or gums;
    h. Injury to tongue.

Repair of Facial Injury

Repair of facial injuries are secondary to the treatment of any life-threatening problem the injured athlete may have. Soft tissue injuries can usually be managed without jeopardizing the seriously injured athlete. If necessary, soft tissue injury can wait for repair up to 24 hours without compromising the final result, providing bleeding has been controlled, and the wound has been properly cleansed and dressed.

Reduction and fixation of facial bone fractures rarely need to be considered an emergency. Conditions should be as nearly ideal as possible before attempting any but the simplest type of reduction. Facial bone fractures become more difficult to reduce once healing has begun between the fracture fragments. From a practical standpoint, most facial bone fractures can be readily reduced within a two week period following injury, except in young children, when reduction should be attempted in seven to ten days due to accelerated healing at these ages. In any case, suspected facial fractures should be referred to a physician for diagnosis and treatment.

Chapter XIV

Dental Injuries

Edward G. Burnett, Jr.

Most traumatic dental injuries, whether incurred during a sports activity or any other activity, are relatively minor. The majority of these are cracked and chipped teeth. This chapter will consider some epidemiologic facts about traumatic dental injuries, on-site treatment procedures which can be handled by parents or coaches, and a brief discussion of the importance of using mouth protectors for prevention of dental injuries.

Epidemiology

It appears that in childhood there are times during which dental injuries are more likely to occur. The first peak seems to be from ages two to five, when the child is learning to walk and then run, but lacks the coordination to do so safely. The next most likely age range seems to be between eight and twelve, coinciding with participation in sports, bicycling, skateboarding, and playground activities. Dental research indicates that by the completion of high school, one of every three boys, and one of every four girls, will have suffered a dental injury. With the recent emphasis on women's athletics, girls are almost as likely to suffer dental injuries as are boys.

Research also indicates that about 90 percent of all traumatic dental injuries are chipped teeth, with the remainder being severe tooth crown fractures which expose the pulp of the tooth, and tooth displacement or avulsion. It is also quite common to find lip and gingival (gum) lacerations with any traumatic dental injury, no matter how minor. Fractured jaws and fractured posterior teeth are relatively uncommon findings.

It appears that the maxillary (upper) incisors, particularly the maxillary central incisors, are the most prone to injury. The vulnerability and severity of injury increases dramatically as protrusion of these incisors is evidenced. Maxillary lateral incisors, followed by mandibular (lower) central and lateral incisors are the next most vulnerable. Posterior teeth are rarely injured unless the force of the blow received is from under the chin or jaw.

Treatment

It is important to realize that any traumatic dental injury, no matter how seemingly inconsequential, should be evaluated by a dentist. It is perhaps more important to realize that any dental injury can occur simultaneously with other head, neck, and facial injuries, thus necessitating careful neurologic evaluation.

Most of the treatment of dental injuries, other than general first aid measures, is beyond the scope of non-dental personnel. Discussion of treatment procedures will, therefore, be confined to the immediate on-site treatment necessary in cases of displaced teeth.

Displaced teeth may be divided into three categories; subluxation (tooth displacement less than 5mm), partial avulsion (displacement more than 5mm), and avulsion (tooth out of its socket). Subluxations may go unnoticed by non-dental personnel. However, if noticed, the tooth should be repositioned, if possible. Partial avulsions will probably be evident, and again the treatment involves repositioning the tooth as soon as possible. In cases of permanent tooth avulsion, time is of the utmost importance. The chances of successful replantation are best if the tooth can be replanted within 30 minutes. The prognosis of the case dramatically decreases as extraoral time increases. In situations where the tooth has just been avulsed (knocked out) and can be found, the following procedure is recommended. If the tooth is dirty, it should be held by the crown portion, and gently rinsed under tap water, taking care not to scrub the tooth. The tooth should then be gently placed back into the socket, and held there by the patient or parent while being transported to the dentist. If tooth replantation at the site is not possible (heavy bleeding, patient fear, etc.), the tooth should be carried to the dentist's office in a container of milk, saline (salt water) solution, or water. Milk is the preferred medium of transportation. If milk, saline solution, or water is not available, and the athlete is not medically impaired, the tooth can be carried to the dentist's office in the patient's buccal vestibule (between the cheek and gum).

Mouth Protectors (Mouth Guards)

Research has shown conclusively that oral injuries are drastically reduced during athletics when mouth guards are worn. Prior to the use of face protectors and mouth guards, about 50 percent of all football injuries were oral injuries. Now this percentage has been reportedly reduced to as low as .5 percent. It is because of this effective reduction in dental injuries that most high schools adopted a mandatory mouth guard program in 1962, and the National Collegiate Athletic Association implemented a similar rule in 1973. In addition to preventing dental injuries, it has been demonstrated that mouth guards may afford protection against concussions and neck injuries. Most of the research on mouth protection devices has been confined to the sports of football and boxing where these devices have been in use the longest. However, the use of mouth protectors in other sports such as baseball, basketball, ice hockey, field hockey, lacrosse, wrestling, rugby, soccer, gymnastics, karate, and judo is strongly recommended.

A satisfactory mouth guard should have some specific properties. It must have sufficient body so that sharply localized blows can be spread over a considerable area of the teeth and maxilla, yet be resilient enough to allow the energy from these blows to be absorbed and the guard to return to its original shape. It should be smooth, retentive, tasteless, odorless, and, when in use, should not impede speech or breathing, or otherwise be uncomfortable in the mouth. In addition, it should be durable, easy to fabricate, and relatively inexpensive.

Mouth guards generally fall into one of three categories based upon the different methods of fabrication, player acceptance (i.e., fit, comfort, etc.), cost, and degree of protection. Stock, unfitted mouth guards are considered the least desirable form of mouth protectors because of poor fit and retention, thus poor player acceptance. However, this type does offer some protection, and is inexpensive.

Custom-fitted mouth guards are most likely to be accepted by the athlete in terms of fit and comfort. They offer the best protection, but are the most expensive and most difficult to fabricate. These protectors are made from casts of the athlete's mouth, utilizing a procedure much like that used in constructing dentures.

The third type may be called mouth-formed protectors. These guards are positioned in an athlete's mouth, and permitted to mold to the player's teeth by thermosetting or chemosetting. When properly fitted, this type of mouth protector has a high level of acceptance while affording adequate protection and cost effectiveness. Many local dental organizations and societies have active programs to aid school and youth sports programs in utilization of this type of protector for their athletes. Information on such programs may sometimes be obtained by contacting the local dental society.

In conclusion, mouth protectors continue to be the most effective method of preventing traumatic dental injuries, and their use should be advocated by all coaches and parents involved with any youth sports program.

Chapter XV

Eye Injuries

M. Bruce Shields and John E. Bourgeois

Sports injuries of the eye and adjacent structures are relatively common, despite the protective mechanisms of the visual system. Prompt recognition and correct initial management of eye injuries by players, coaches, parents, or others who happen to be the first on the scene can significantly reduce ocular morbidity and blindness. This chapter provides information relative to the appropriate initial care of ocular sports injuries.

Ocular Anatomy

Recognition and appropriate emergency management of eye injuries requires at least a fundamental knowledge of ocular and orbital anatomy. The eye itself is spherical and approximately 2.5 cm. in diameter. This shape is maintained by two fluids within the eye; the aqueous humor anteriorly, and the jelly-like vitreous posteriorly. The normal cornea is clear, which allows light to enter the eye. The sclera extends from the cornea backwards to the optic nerve, and is made of tough connective tissue, which gives it an opaque, white appearance. Within the eye, the iris is situated behind the cornea, and is separated from the latter structure by the aqueous. The color of this diaphragm determines whether a person has blue, green, or brown eyes. The central opening in the iris is called the pupil. The muscles in the iris, by constricting and relaxing, control the size of the pupil, which thereby regulates the amount of light entering the eye. The lens is located behind the iris and is normally clear. Light entering the eye is focused by the cornea and lens onto the light sensitive retina in the back of the eye. The retina contains layers of cells which transform light images into electrical impulses which are carried by the optic nerve to the brain for interpretation.

The eye is protected in front by the eyelids and lashes. Reflex closure of the lids serves as an important protective mechanism. The inner portion of the eyelids is covered by a layer of mucous membrane called the conjunctiva, which extends onto the front of the eye, covering the anterior sclera up to the cornea. This membrane contains the blood vessels which frequently dilate or even rupture and bleed with ocular irritation or injury.

The eye is surrounded by a bony orbit, which provides protection on the sides the behind the globe. Muscles extend from these bones to the sclera to move the eye. Although the bony orbit protects the eye from many injuries, orbital fractures are not uncommon, and frequently interfere with eye movement.

Prevention of Ocular Injuries

Since 1973, the number of eye injuries related to sports products has risen by nearly 60%. The National Society to Prevent Blindness estimates that 90% of the sports-related eye injuries are preventable. Unfortunately, children 5-14 years of age suffer nearly one-third of all sports and recreation-related eye injuries.

Street wear spectacles with either plastic or glass lenses do not offer adequate eye protection in any sport which can involve blows to the face with a ball, racquet, bat, fist, elbow, or any other object. This includes tennis and badminton. If the athlete insists on wearing street wear spectacles only, then plastic lenses are safer than glass.

Contact lenses offer no eye protection and indeed hard contact lenses place the athlete at greater risk of injury. Contact lens wearers should utilize the same protective equipment as described above for players who do not wear contact lenses.

It is especially dangerous for one-eyed children to play collision or contact sports. If participation is allowed in sports such as football, hockey, field hockey, or lacrosse, safety glasses should be worn beneath the helmet-face mask combinations. A fine mesh wire hockey face shield should be used instead of the bar-type football face mask. Ideally, one-eyed children should not participate in racquet sports or handball. However, if participation is allowed, the safety equipment mentioned previously for racquet sports should be utilized.

Parents, coaches, and supervisors can greatly reduce the number of eye injuries in children by insisting that proper eye protection devices be utilized in sports. The following table outlines the recommended levels of protection for various sports:

Recommended Levels of Eye Protection for Sports Activities

COLLISION SPORTS

Certified helmet plus face mask designed for the sport
1. For hockey, face mask must have Hockey Equipment Certification Council (HECC) certification;
2. For football, full face mask rather than single bar;
3. For athletes with only one functional eye, an ASTM F 803 eye protector should be worn in addition to a face mask.

OTHER SPORTS WITH POTENTIAL FOR BALL, STICK, RACQUET OR BODY CONTACT

Safest: 1. Eye protector which meets ASTM F 803 Standard specifications;

Adequate: 2. Polycarbonate industrial safety lenses (ANSI Z 87.1) mounted in industrial frame;

                3. For tennis and badminton, polycarbonate lenses in sturdy streetwear frame.

Eye Protection Devices Not Recommended For Athletes

1. Street wear eyeglasses with glass or ordinary plastic lenses (These pose a definite hazard of eye laceration if struck with force);
2. Contact lenses without an eye protector in sports which require eye protection (contact lenses offer no protection);
3. Lensless eye protectors for racquet sports (These offer no significant protection);
4. Bare eyes in sports which require eye protection.

Note: Protective devices decrease, but do not eliminate the chance of injury. The above recommendations are subject to change pending future data.

From Vinger, Paul F. "Sports-Related Eye Injury: A Preventable Problem", Survey of Ophthalmology, 25:1, 1980. Modified and reprinted with permission.

Initial Management of Ocular Injuries

Proper initial management of eye injuries on the playing field or court not only can help relieve the pain of the victim, but can help to prevent visual loss. Certain general principles should be observed whenever one examines an eye: 1) Avoid examining an eye with dirty hands. When it is not possible to wash the hands first, place the fingers only on the eyelids, well away from the lid margins. 2) Be careful, gentle, and thorough, since an examination that is too hasty or rigorous can worsen the injury. 3) Never exert pressure on an injured eye, because a laceration or rupture may be present. 4) Ask the victim if his/her vision is impaired, since reduced vision always implies sufficient injury to require professional care.

Foreign Body Injuries. Foreign bodies of many types and sizes (dirt, grass, etc.) can enter the eye during sports activities. They frequently lodge between the lid and globe, especially under the upper lid. The injured person will experience a scratchy sensation with increased tearing, and the eye will appear red and irritated as the conjunctival vessels dilate. Do not allow the victim to rub his/her eyes, as this may push the foreign body into the tissues, and abrade the cornea. To inspect the eye for a foreign body, first gently pull down the lower lid, and ask the patient to look up. Foreign matter visualized between the lower eyelid and globe should be gently wiped away with a cotton-tipped applicator, or irrigated away with appropriate balanced salt solutions. If commercial solutions for irrigating the eye are not available, clean tap water may be used.

To thoroughly examine the under-surface of the upper eyelid for a foreign body, the upper lid must be everted. This maneuver requires a cotton-tipped applicator or a similar small, rod-shaped instrument, such as a match stick. First, have the individual look down at his/her feet. Then, grasp the lashes of the upper lid between your thumb and forefinger, and gently pull the lid away from the globe. Now, place the smooth stick portion of the instrument horizontally along the upper outer surface of the upper lid, and pull the lid up and over the stick, thereby exposing the underside of the lid. Gently remove any visible foreign body with a clean cotton-tipped applicator or with irrigation. Dust or other matter which is too small to remove with a cotton swab must be irrigated.

If a foreign body is seen to be lodged in the cornea, do not try to remove it. The eye should be gently patched, and the individual taken to a physician immediately. Whenever an ocular injury is sufficient to require medical attention, it is best to have the patient seen by an opthalmologist, a doctor of medicine who specializes in the medical and surgical care of the eye. When this is not possible, an emergency room physician or other doctor should be sought.

A larger foreign body can become imbedded in the globe. Do not try to remove it. If possible, the injured eye should be covered with a paper cup and tape, taking care not to dislodge the foreign object. Any pressure on the eye, even by the eyelids or a gentle patch, may force the foreign body farther into the eye. If no materials are available to serve as a protective canopy, then transport the individual immediately to medical care, being careful not to bump the impacted object. Calm reassurance is also needed.

In some sports situations, especially when guns are involved, a high-velocity foreign body may completely penetrate the front of the eye, and lodge in the back of the globe or in the orbit. Such injuries require immediate attention by an opthalmologist. Occasionally, the site of entry is so small that the presence of such an intraocular foreign body is missed. Therefore, whenever there is a question of such an injury, immediate medical evaluation should be sought.

Corneal Abrasions and Lacerations. Frequently, an object (finger, racquet, etc.) can strike the front of the eye, and cause a corneal abrasion. A portion of the cornea is stripped of its outer layer of cells by such an injury, thereby exposing raw nerve endings to the external environment. Such an injury will be accompanied by intense pain, redness, tearing, light sensitivity, foreign body sensation, and blurred vision. A corneal abrasion may not be apparent by gross examination, but the diagnosis can usually be made on the basis of the aforementioned signs and symptoms. One should gently open the lids, and examine the eyeball for an obvious cut on the cornea or a foreign body. If neither is found, gently patch the injured eye, and transport the patient to appropriate medical care. If the cornea or sclera is noted to be lacerated, do not search further for a foreign body. Specifically, do not evert the lid, and do not allow pressure to be exerted on the globe. Gently cover the eye with a clean dressing, and immediately transport the victim to medical care.

Injuries to the Eyelid and Surrounding Structures. Trauma to the eyelids can result in either a contusion injury (bruise) or laceration.

67

Contusion injuries to the lids result in swelling and redness as the blood vessels in the lids rupture (a black eye). Such injury to the lids in and of itself is not serious, since swelling and blood will absorb spontaneously within several weeks. However, any injury significant enough to cause a contusion injury to the lids warrants examination by an opthalmologist within 24 hours, or immediately if visual loss is noted. Such examination is necessary because internal ocular structures may also have been damaged which are not apparent with casual external inspection.

Lacerations of the lid usually bleed profusely because of their rich blood supply. As in the case of contusion injuries to the eyelids, it is important to carefully look for evidence of damage to the eyeball itself. Specifically, one should check for injuries to the cornea or sclera, blood behind the cornea, and reduced vision. If the eyeball itself does not appear to be injured, the bleeding from the lids can usually be controlled by direct pressure over a clean bandage. Never apply pressure to the eye if the globe appears damaged, since ocular fluids and other contents might be forced out, causing irreparable damage. If the eye does appear to be injured, merely cover both eyes gently with a clean bandage, and rapidly transport the victim to medical care.

If an individual complains of double vision when looking in any direction following an ocular injury, he/she should be seen immediately by his/her physician, since the thin bones of the orbit may have been broken, thereby entrapping the muscles which move the eye. This condition may be manifested by the inability of the injured eye to move parallel with the fellow eye and/or by the injured eye sinking backward into its orbit.

Extrusion of Globe. Occasionally, trauma may be severe enough to cause extrusion of an eyeball. Do not attempt to push the eye back into its socket. The eye should gently be covered with moist gauze, and the patient should be carefully transported on his/her back to an emergency room.

Chapter XVI

Head and Neck Injuries

J.M. McWhorter

Every year in the United States, needless deaths and severe neurological injuries occur among our younger population as a result of athletic participation. While most of these injuries occur during participation in contact sports, no athletic endeavor is risk-free with respect to head and/ or spinal cord injury. Perhaps the most logical way to approach this problem is by preventing situations during athletic participation in which one is most apt to sustain a head or spinal cord injury.

Protective Equipment

Over the years, equipment manufacturers have upgraded their products to offer maximum protection to the head and spinal cord. However, if the equipment is not fitted to the individual, some elements of its protective purpose are eliminated. Equipment, particularly helmets used in football, baseball, and hockey must be well matched to the athlete to provide the utmost in protection from head injuries. If the protective equipment does not fit well, then the protection that equipment affords is of little value.

Instruction and Supervision

Youngsters who are going to participate in sports activities, particularly contact sports, should be trained in the essentials of that sport. They should be taught the proper way to block and tackle, so that the head and neck are properly protected during such maneuvers. They should be physically fit, and a preparticipation physical examination is mandatory. Lastly, in all organized sports there should be adequate supervision so that the risks of head and spinal cord injuries are minimized.

Injury Recognition and Management

This year throughout the United States, there will be more than 50,000 concussions sustained by high school football players. Therefore, it is necessary for coaches and trainers to know how to correctly assess head and neck injuries on the playing field. In evaluating a player on the football field, soccer field, or basketball court with a suspected head or cervical spine injury (the differentiation between the two is often difficult), the first step is to check the player's level of consciousness. Is the player awake and alert? Is he/she able to answer simple questions? Is he/she complaining of numbness or tingling in his/her hands and/or feet? Are his/her pupils equal, and can he/she look to the right and left when told to do so? The athlete should not be moved during this time, and particularly not the head or neck. If he/she is wearing a helmet, it is imperative that the helmet not be removed. This cannot be stressed too strongly since, in actuality, when a player is injured, the first thing one may tend to do when examining the athlete is to take the helmet off. In removing the helmet, one necessarily moves the neck, which may lead to damage to the spinal cord if there is a spine injury.

The helmet can be used, if necessary, as a traction device if a neck injury has occurred. One can use the helmet to provide stability and traction on the patient's head and neck while the player is being moved onto a stretcher. If the facemask does not snap off, bolt cutters may be used to cut it off. If the athlete complains of neck pain, it should be assumed that there has been a serious injury to the spine, and the athlete should be examined by a physician and have x-rays of the neck.

Common Head Injuries

The most common cause of death in athletes involved in contact sports is bleeding inside the head. Skull fractures in contact sports are much rarer now because of the greater protective capabilities of helmets. However, they may still occur, particularly in those athletes that are struck by a baseball or bat or collide with another player. The only way to be sure that a skull fracture has not occurred following a severe blow to the head is to obtain x-rays of the head.

An athlete who receives a blow to the head of such severity that he/she becomes unconscious is another story. This person should be examined by a physician right away, no matter how brief the period of unconsciousness. In contact sports particularly, a player is too often struck on the head, becomes unconscious briefly, sits on the bench for a short time, and then returns to play. After the game is over, he/she returns home not feeling well, complaining of headache, perhaps nausea or vomiting, goes to sleep, and later when someone tries to awaken him/her, he/she is found to be unconscious. In all likelihood, he/she has a serious problem inside the skull, and is in serious condition. Any athlete who sustains a blow to the head, has a brief period of unconsciousness, and becomes alert and feels fine, should be checked by a physician. If found to be normal, he/she should be observed closely by his/her parents for at least twenty four hours after the injury. Any player who loses consciousness, even briefly, should not return to play during that day.

The most common problem developing in the head from a head injury is a blood clot which forms over the surface of the brain. Most athletes who have a head injury severe enough to cause a potentially lethal problem will have a brief period of unconsciousness, after which they may awaken and appear perfectly normal. They may complain of headache, possibly some nausea or vomiting, and become progressively more sleepy. These youngsters should be evaluated immediately. Those athletes who have had a severe head injury or spine injury, or who have had repeated concussions, should be permanently eliminated from participation in contact sports.

As a "rule of thumb", any athlete who has had a head injury or spine injury, no matter how minor, should be evaluated by a physician at the first opportunity. Parents and coaches should recognize that it is much safer to stop an athlete's participation in a particular sport until he/she is cleared by a physician.

It is important to remember that ...
1. Any blow to the head is potentially serious, and should not be taken lightly with such trite phrases as "The kid just got his bell rung; he'll be OK," or "She's OK; only a little dazed."
2. If a head and/or neck injury is suspected, do not move the injured athlete. Call for emergency medical services. The game can wait!
3. The following signs may indicate the existence of a serious head and/ or neck injury:
   a. Player remains unconscious;
   b. Player complains of severe headache and/or neck pain;
   c. Player cannot move arms or legs;
   d. Convulsions;
   e. Blurred vision, restless, agitated, staggers, appears "dopey", confused;
   f. Severe nausea and/or vomiting;
   g. Drainage of either blood or clear fluid from either ears or nose.

Chapter XVII

Chest and Abdominal Injuries

James H. Manly, Jr.

Everyone familiar with sports tends to think of injuries in terms of injured knees, sprained ankles, broken bones, or injuries of the head and neck. These are all too frequently seen on the practice or playing field or on television presentations. Often more mysterious and worrisome to coaches, parents, young athletes, and spectators are injuries to the chest and abdomen. For those interested in and charged with a degree of responsibility for the health and well-being of young athletes, it is important to gain at least a minimal knowledge of the organs which reside within the chest and abdomen which may be injured or cause distressing symptoms during sports activity.

Chest and Abdominal Anatomy

The chest and abdomen may be considered as one large cavity divided into upper and lower halves by a sheet of muscle called the diaphragm. The upper half (chest) contains the heart and lungs. Every adult should know that the heart pumps out blood to the rest of the body. Actually the right half of the heart pumps blood to the lungs, and the left side pumps blood returning from the lungs to the rest of the body. The reason for pumping blood to the lungs is to exchange carbon dioxide for oxygen in the red blood cells.

We all know that the increased physical activity of sports causes us to breathe more vigorously, and the reason for this is that there is a greater need to rapidly exchange carbon dioxide for oxygen. The lungs are like large sponges with all of the air cells connected to a single windpipe. When we breathe in, the oxygen in the air passes through the windpipe to the further most parts of the spongy lungs, and passes through the thin walls of the small air tubes to exchange places with carbon dioxide which is being carried by the hemoglobin in the red blood cells.

All body tissues use oxygen to produce energy for activity in much the same way that a burning log must have oxygen, or it cannot continue to burn. Basically the substances used by the body for energy are carbohydrates (sugar) and fats. When these are "burned" to produce aerobic (with oxygen) energy, carbon dioxide is produced, and oxygen is diminished. This, therefore, requires that the carbon dioxide be taken to the lungs for exchange for new oxygen supplies. If this does not occur, the individual would get into great difficulty. It follows, therefore, that any problem that obstructs the flow of air down the windpipe, or which interferes with the exchange function of the lungs is going to severely affect an athlete.

The lower half of the body cavity (abdomen) contains a variety of important organs including the liver, pancreas, spleen, kidneys, stomach, and upper intestine. In the female, the abdomen is also the location of the reproductive organs. The abdominal organs are responsible for a wide variety of vital functions. Therefore, injuries to the abdomen are potentially serious, and occasionally life-threatening.

The organs of the chest are rather well protected by the twelve ribs and heavy muscles about the chest, shoulders, and upper abdomen. The abdominal organs, on the other hand, are less well protected, and, therefore, more vulnerable to injury.

Common Injuries

The most common chest injuries are simply having the breath knocked out and direct blows to the ribs resulting in contusions and/or fractures.

"Wind Knocked Out". When one has the "wind knocked out", it may have come from a blow to the abdomen, chest, or back. The lungs are forcibly compressed, and a momentary shock to the breathing mechanism takes place. Apparently the small air spaces have trouble refilling, so the most important thing to do is reassure the athlete, and it will take care of itself. Almost anything, or nothing, you do will eventually bring about relief. However, it is important to be certain that nothing is obstructing the air flow of the windpipe. This is especially important if the athlete becomes somewhat blue (cyanotic). In this case, see if a doctor is available immediately, or contact emergency medical services as soon as possible.

Rib Fracture. In case of suspected rib fracture, there is general pain in the area. Bruises of the rib or cartilage can be very painful. If one places the hands on the sides of the chest and compresses the rib cage, a fractured rib

73

will be manifested by a sharply localized, severe pain at the fracture site. Also, front and back compression is useful in making this determination. A fractured rib will often produce sharply localized pain when the athlete takes a deep breath. If one decides that a rib is cracked or broken, a pressure dressing with sponge pad over the suspected fracture site may give relief. Occasionally, a slightly cracked rib in a particular athlete may permit resumption of activity. However, heavily padding a wide area and a pressure dressing must be employed. Rib fractures are usually painful for two to four weeks. A physician should decide when the athlete may return to participation.

Kidney Injuries. The kidneys are the most frequently injured of the intra-abdominal organs, and, like all abdominal injuries, result from rather violent compression such as direct blows which squeeze the organ against some rigid structure such as the backbone or ribs. Happily, in the case of the kidneys, most of the injuries represent simple bruising or very slight lacerations which do not require surgical exploration. However, such determinations should be made by a physician. The symptoms of kidney injury are usually those of pain in the abdomen and/or pain in the back across the lower ribs. Usually, with the first passing of urine, the urine contains some blood, and may be identified by appearing somewhat smoky or actually blood-tinged. Any athlete with these symptoms should be evaluated by a physician.

Spleen injuries. Injuries to the spleen are the next most common of the serious abdominal injuries. The spleen rests high up under the diaphragm on the left side, and is protected all around except in the pit of the stomach area. This protection is provided by the backbone, ribs, stomach, and diaphragm. Tears of the spleen attachments or breaks in the fragile splenic tissue result in bleeding to varying degrees. The ribs are flexible in youngsters, and a blow over the ribs on the left side can permit the ribs to strike the spleen without fracturing the ribs. Symptoms of spleen injury are similar to having the "breath knocked out", along with pain in the left upper abdomen which spreads along the left side of the abdomen, pain in the shoulder, and tenderness on the left side of the neck. The athlete may appear sweaty and pale with cool skin (signs of shock). Other signs (which you may see and/or feel) include tightness of the muscles in the area of the left upper abdomen which resists pressure of the hands to the tender area. Usually there is grunting breathing, and a desire not to move or be moved.

74

All of these are signs of irritation of the delicate peritoneal membrane which lines the abdominal cavity, and which covers most of the organs. Bleeding from a badly torn spleen can be very vigorous, and immediate transfer to the hospital is necessary. Spleens which are enlarged by various diseases are much more easily injured than normal-sized spleens. In youngsters, mononucleosis ("kissing disease") is relatively common, and often causes enlargement of the spleen, and, more importantly, may result in a spleen which is extremely fragile and easily torn. One study determined that approximately one-half of all splenic injuries occur in youngsters with mononucleosis. All spleen injuries require physician evaluation and care, and most result in surgical treatment.

Pancreas Injuries. The pancreas lies across the backbone at about the level of the "solar plexus", which is approximately half way between the navel and the lower end of the breastbone. This relatively unprotected area permits hard blows to compress the pancreas against the backbone, often producing injury. Usually injuries to the pancreas are mild, and make the athlete sick, with enough pain to stop sport participation for a few days. Rarely are these injuries serious enough to require hospitalization and treatment. Pain, tenderness, and perhaps nausea and vomiting are the most common symptoms. Suspected pancreatic injuries should be referred to a physician for evaluation.

Liver Injuries. Liver injuries are more rare than those discussed previously. Rarely is the liver torn enough to produce internal bleeding. However, the same basic symptoms and signs as those associated with spleen injury may be present, except that such symptoms will occur on the right side of the abdomen. Suspected liver injuries should be referred to a physician for evaluation.

Playing During Illness

Young athletes will often attempt to participate in practice or games when they are otherwise ill. Careful observation of the youngster's behavior, color, and performance will frequently indicate that he/she is not completely well. Such youngsters should be carefully questioned with regard to upset stomach, sore throat, headache, fever, aches and pains, and just plain "feeling bad". If this is the case, the young athlete should not be permitted to participate. A healthy "second stringer" can usually play better than a sick "first stringer". Moreover, the sick or injured athlete is more prone to further injury or illness than a healthy one.

It is important to note that many athletes go on the field with various diseases such as colds, upset stomachs, diarrhea, etc., and do not report this to coaches or parents, feeling that it is simply due to pregame jitters. During the game, however, these symptoms may intensify, producing severe pain in the chest, shortness of breath, and/or abdominal cramping. In case of increasing symptoms, the athlete may be in extreme distress. It is important to carefully question the athlete to determine if the symptoms are the result of an abdominal blow received in the game or non-injury effects of an existing sickness.

Most often an athlete who suffers a blow to the chest or abdomen will have the symptoms disappear fairly quickly. However, if the cause of the symptoms is viral disease of the intestine or other disease-related problem, the symptoms frequently do not go away quickly, but continue to worsen with time. Whatever the suspected cause, the athlete who suffers from such symptoms should be withdrawn from sport participation, and referred to a physician for evaluation and care.

Chapter XVIII

Upper Extremity Injuries

John A. King

Injuries to the upper extremity are common in sports. Many extremity injuries in children may be of the same nature as in an adult. However, differences in structure and physical ability exist, making certain injuries specific to the child or adolescent.

Fortunately, the vast majority of extremity injuries are minor. Only approximately 5% of sports injuries are fractures. Coaches and parents have a large responsibility to not only care for serious injuries, but to spot early signs of physical problems which are less severe. Because the pain is not intense, the athlete may ignore the problem leading to chronic conditions such as overuse syndromes. Proper equipment, training, and coaching are all part of injury prevention. More injuries occur in free play than in organized team sports. Therefore, good supervision can prevent many needless injuries.

The young athlete is not merely a smaller version of an adult. Young bones possess many growth plates. These regions are usually located near the joints, and are necessary for the limbs to grow longer. Because the growth plate is not yet bone, it represents a potential site for a type of injury not found in adults. These growth centers may be injured not only by a traumatic event, but also by overuse or repetitive activity.

Shoulder and Upper Arm Injuries

The shoulder girdle is comprised of the scapula (shoulder blade), the clavicle (collar bone), and the humerus (upper arm bone). The bones form the shoulder joint, and are held together by ligaments. The nerves and blood vessels that supply the upper extremity pass the shoulder in the axilla (arm pit). Muscles and tendons attach to the bones, and cause movement at the joint. All these structures may be involved in injury.

"Burners". "Burners" (or "stingers") usually occur when there is a direct blow to the top of the shoulder as would occur when blocking or tackling in football. This injury is caused by an instantaneous stretch of the nerves as they exit the neck and cross the shoulder joint, rendering the upper extremity weak, numb, and often painful — usually momentarily. If symptoms persist, or involve both upper extremities simultaneously, the athlete should not be allowed to return to play, and should be seen by a physician.

Contusions. Contusions (bruises) can occur anywhere in the upper extremity. If a severe bruise occurs to the muscles of the upper arm, bleeding into the muscle may result in calcification leading to a condition known as myositis ossificans (calcium deposit). This usually occurs if the athlete returns to participation, and the area is reinjured. If the bruise is not severe, and the athlete plans to compete, the arm should be padded to prevent reinjury. If pain or swelling is dramatic, and range of motion at the elbow is limited, the athlete should be withheld from competition. Rest is required until the signs are resolved.

Sprains. Sprains involve injury to the supporting ligaments around a joint. At the shoulder these may involve the acromioclavicular joint or shoulder joint. The acromioclavicular joint resides at the distal (outer) end of the clavicle above the shoulder joint. Injury usually occurs from a fall on the point of the shoulder, and may result in pain and a variable degree of deformity above the shoulder.

Sprains of the shoulder joint (between the humerus and scapula) involve dislocations and subluxations. Dislocations represent a complete separation of the joint with deformity, and the inability to move the shoulder. Shoulder ligaments are usually torn. With subluxation, a partial separation of the shoulder joint occurs.

Deformity is not usually produced, but the pain may be as severe as with dislocation. Ligaments are not always torn, but may be rendered incompetent. Because neurovascular structures pass beneath the shoulder, nerve damage may occur. An athlete with a sprain or dislocation should not be allowed to return to participation if the pain persists or deformity is present. Reduction of a dislocation (putting it back in place) should not be attempted because a fracture may be present. Immediate medical attention should be sought. If the injury is recurrent, surgery may be needed to stabilize the joint.

Fractures. The clavicle is the most frequently fractured bone in small children. Eighty percent occur in the midportion of the bone. Pain, swelling, and deformity are generally present. Fractures may occur involving the upper growth plate of the humerus. These manifest the same signs as shoulder subluxation/dislocation. Fractures involving the shaft (midportion) of the humerus are less common in children than in adults, if growth plates remain open. In addition to pain and deformity, crepitation (a grating sensation at the fracture site) may be detected. Any suspected serious injury to the shoulder should be immobilized by strapping the arm and forearm to the body. Some shoulder dislocations may cause the upper arm to be positioned away from the body. Immobilization should be in the position of greatest comfort. Prompt medical attention should be sought.

Elbow and Forearm Injuries

The elbow is composed of the lower end of the humerus, and the upper end of the radius and ulna (forearm bones). Ligaments, muscles, and the bony structure stabilize this joint. Six growth centers comprise the elbow, making this joint susceptible to injury in young athletes.

Contusions/Abrasions. The elbow is highly susceptible to contusions (bruises) and abrasions (scrapes). Abrasions should be cleaned thoroughly, and a sterile dressing applied. If the participant is to return to activity, the area should be padded well until the area heals.

Fractures. Fractures to the elbow can involve the growth centers if they remain open. Pain, swelling, and deformity can result. There is usually inability to bend or straighten the elbow fully. Dislocations may also occur. This may or may not be associated with a fracture. Nerve and blood vessels across the joint are at risk with severe injury because of the anatomy of the elbow. Signs of numbness, lack of pulse, or pallor in the forearm or hand make these injuries an extreme emergency, requiring immediate medical attention. The joint, arm, and forearm should be splinted, and prompt medical attention should be sought.

The forearm is composed of two bones, the radius and the ulna. Fractures cause pain and deformity. If severe, crepitation may be present. The elbow, forearm, and wrist should be splinted, and medical advise sought.

Wrist and Hand Injuries

The wrist and hand are made up of numerous bones. The muscles of the forearm form tendons which flex and extend the wrist and fingers. Tendons, as well as nerves and blood vessels are very superficial structures in this region. If profuse bleeding occurs, a blood vessel may have been lacerated. Direct pressure should be applied with a clean cloth, and the participant transported to a medical facility. Deep lacerations may also injure tendons. Motion of one or more fingers may be lost.

Avulsions. Tendon avulsions may also occur if a tendon is torn from its bony attachment on the finger. This may result in loss of motion (flexion or extension) of a digit. Avulsions usually involve the distal (end) joint of a digit. Many times this occurs with tackling a runner when grabbing the shirt. Medical treatment is required.

Fractures. Wrist fractures usually occur from a fall on an outstretched hand. Pain, swelling, and, occasionally, deformity occur. It is a myth that the wrist and/or digits cannot be moved if a fracture is present. If fracture is suspected, the wrist and forearm should be splinted, and the athlete taken to a medical facility.

Fractures and dislocations of the digits are fairly common. Pain, deformity, and immobility frequently occur. The deformity should not be reduced on the playing field by an untrained person because it is often difficult to determine if the injury is a fracture or a dislocation. Attempts to reduce a fracture may damage other structures. Dislocations that are reduced may correct the deformity, but splinting may be required to prevent later loss of function.

"Skiers' Thumb". Injury to the ligaments at the base of the thumb can occur with stress applied which bends the thumb out away from the hand. This injury has been coined "skiers' thumb" because of its frequent occurrence when falling onto a ski pole held in the hand. Other mechanisms of injury are possible. Extreme swelling and/or looseness at the base of the thumb should be assessed by a physician.

Overuse Syndromes

Once more common in adults than in children, overuse syndromes are becoming more frequent among young athletes. These injuries are not the result of a single traumatic event. Repetitive activity or improper training are frequent causes. Doing too much of one activity over a short period of time, or abrupt changes in training intensity can lead to these injuries. Sport-specific camps are frequently a major contributing factor. The body simply cannot always adjust to six to eight hours of training per day, when it is used to one to two.

Impingement Syndrome. Impingement syndrome in the shoulder produces inflammation of the rotator cuff muscles. This may be caused by repetitive overhead activity, involved in throwing sports, tennis, and swimming. Pain on lifting the arm is the key symptom. In the younger athlete, this may be a sign of shoulder subluxation or instability.

Tendinitis. Tendinitis in the hand or elbow results from microscopic tearing or injury of the tendon, or from inflammation of the tissues surrounding the tendon. "Tennis elbow" is an example, causing pain on the lateral (outside) aspect of the elbow. Improper technique is a primary factor in its development.

Stress Fractures. Stress fractures may be described as injury to bony structures resulting from repetitive activity. In the young athlete, this may occur at the weaker growth plate. These injuries may occur from repetitive throwing frequently seen in young pitchers who throw too many innings in a game, or are not given time enough to rest between games pitched. "Little League shoulder" is a stress fracture of the upper growth plate of the humerus. "Little League elbow" is a stress fracture of one of the growth centers at the elbow. Gymnasts may have similar injuries to the growth plate at the wrist. Permanent damage can result with these injuries if the repetition continues despite pain.

Treatment of overuse syndromes includes rest or immobilization, ice, compression, and elevation. Once symptoms have resolved, return to sports should be slow and staged. The best treatment, of course, is prevention, including correct strengthening and stretching exercises prior to the sport. Proper guidance by adults cannot be over-stressed in the supervision of these special athletes.

Chapter XIX

Lower Extremity Injuries

Timothy N. Taft

The lower extremities are the most commonly injured parts of the body involved in training and competition. Most problems result from a single identifiable injury. There are, however, an increasing number of conditions due to overuse, abuse, or excessive and repetitive stress. The injuries caused by the cumulative effect of multiple small (often unrecognized) injuries can be just as devastating as one single major trauma.

The prevention of injuries should be a major goal of anyone responsible for supervising athletic activities. The single major injury is best prevented by a combination of proper equipment and facilities, competent coaching, and a well designed conditioning program. The overuse syndromes are best prevented by a conditioning program which allows the athlete to gradually increase strength and endurance, and which avoids sudden changes in the training regimen.

Such a program requires anticipation of the season, and must be interspersed with resting times so the tissues can recover from athletic stress. The best acute management of athletic injuries is with a combination of ice, compression, elevation, and immobilization. Ice will help diminish swelling and partially anesthetize the injured part, thus making the patient more comfortable. Compression and elevation will help reduce swelling. Immobilization helps prevent additional injury, and makes the patient more comfortable. These four techniques are beneficial for most athletic injuries.

Pelvis and Hip Injuries
The hip joint is formed by an articulation between the femur (thigh bone) and pelvis. It is a ball and socket joint with the head of the femur (ball) seated deeply within the acetabulum (socket) on the pelvis. Injuries to the hip joint itself are relatively uncommon.

Slipped Capital Femoral Epiphysis. This injury is rare, but requires prompt surgery if it occurs. The head of the femur may separate from its shaft at the cartilage growth plate. The cartilagenous plate is not as strong as the surrounding bone, and thus more susceptible to stress. This injury usually occurs in overweight children between the ages of 11 and 13, and the mechanism is a sudden rotational stress to the hip. The child complains of inability to move the hip, and has severe pain in the groin. Occasionally the athlete may complain of thigh or knee pain, rather than hip pain. Anytime a child complains of thigh or knee pain, one must remember that hip injuries often cause thigh and knee pain. The patient with this injury should be promptly transported by stretcher to a physician. Occasionally, this slipping occurs gradually, and any child who complains of persistent groin, thigh, or knee pain should be evaluated by a physician.

Hip Pointer. A direct blow to the iliac crest (hip bone) may cause blood to accumulate beneath the periosteum, which is the outer covering of the bone. This injury occurs when a hard, blunt object strikes directly on the iliac crest. The patient complains of severe pain directly at the site of the blow, and there is marked point tenderness. This is not a particularly serious injury, but one which causes great pain for seven to ten days. Occasionally it is necessary to withdraw the blood from the hematoma, but time and ice packs will usually alleviate the symptoms. Hip pointers are best prevented by protective padding.

Thigh Injuries

Contusions. Contusions (bruises) of the muscles in the thigh are common in contact sports. The muscle can be crushed between the object striking it and the femur. The patient will have point tenderness, and all movement of the contused muscle will be painful. The best immediate treatment is rest, ice, compression, and elevation. Crutches are recommended. Myositis ossificans (calcium deposits within the injured muscle) may occur as a result of this crushing muscle injury. It is more likely to occur if the patient resumes activity while the muscle is still sore. It should be emphasized that all activity following a contusion or strain should be completely within pain tolerance, and any activity that causes pain at the site of injury should be discontinued. Rest is much preferred to "running off" a contusion, because the increased activity will likely cause increased injury to the tissue, and may ultimately delay recovery. All exercise should be conducted without pain. Also, deep muscle bruises should never be massaged since this, too may lead to myositis ossificans. Thigh contusions usually take two to three weeks to recover. If myositis ossificans intervenes, three to five months is generally required before resolution of symptoms.

Strains. Strains (muscle pulls) are uncommon in the pediatric age group, occasionally seen in adolescence, and are reasonably common in young adults. The muscles most commonly affected are those in the groin and the hamstrings in the back of the thigh. The mechanism is a sudden, violent contraction of the muscle such as coming out of the starting blocks in a track meet, or a sudden, unexpected hyperextension of a contracting muscle such as slipping on a wet playing surface. Any number of muscle fibers may be torn, depending upon the severity of the injury. Seldom is the muscle completely torn. The most effective way to deal with muscle strains is to prevent them from occurring. A regular stretching program for muscles at risk will diminish the frequency and severity of acute muscle strains. When a strain does occur, the athlete usually complains of a sudden pulling, stretching, or snapping of the involved muscle. There is point tenderness, and there may be bruising and discoloration because of bleeding into the tissue. There is spasm, and an acutely tender mass where the hemorrhage is developing. If the tear is extensive, weight bearing is impossible because of the extreme pain. Rest, ice, and compression must be immediately instituted. Nowhere in this treatment program is there any room for the deliberate forcing of activity. Despite widespread belief in the athletic world, a muscle pull cannot be "run out". Any attempt to push such an injury inevitably leads to additional tearing of the muscle, and prolongation of the recovery period. Following resolution of the acute symptoms, one should begin a gentle range of motion and activity program. All exercises should be performed painlessly, and any activity which causes pain should be avoided.

Knee Injuries

Collateral Ligament Sprains. The collateral ligaments prevent the knee from bending sideways. The medial (inside) collateral ligament is more commonly injured than the lateral (outside) collateral ligament. The medial ligament is stretched and/or torn by a clipping-type injury. The foot is fixed to the surface, and the player is struck on the lateral side (outside) of the knee. If the pain and tenderness are on the side of the knee which received the blow, the injury is most likely a contusion. If the patient has pain on the other side of the knee, one must suspect a torn ligament. A patient with a torn medial ligament will have pain and tenderness over the inside of the knee, and will often complain that it feels as if the knee wobbles. This injury requires prompt medical attention, and the patient should be transported to a physician after the leg has been immobilized.

Cruciate Ligament Injuries. The cruciate ligaments prevent the tibia (shin bone) from sliding forward and backward at the knee, and they also help control rotation of the tibia on the femur. The anterior cruciate ligament is frequently injured by a hyperextension mechanism, or by twisting the knee when landing awkwardly. The patient usually feels a pop or snap within the knee, and there is often significant swelling within 2 to 3 hours. There may or may not be tenderness around the knee. The patient sometimes complains that the knee feels unstable. Walking and running may cause increased pain and giving way. The pain is located within the knee, and the patient is somewhat vague about localizing it. This injury requires prompt medical attention.

Meniscus Cartilage Tears. There are two menisci within the knee. The medial meniscus on the inside and the lateral meniscus on the outside. The menisci are made of a special type of cartilage, and can be torn by rotating quickly on the weight bearing leg. The menisci are also likely to be torn by full squatting and occasionally by a clipping-type injury. An athlete with a torn meniscus usually feels or hears a pop or snap within the knee, and is unable to completely straighten the knee. There will be pain on the side of the tear. Swelling usually appears within 15 to 20 hours, rather than the two to three hours associated with cruciate tears. Occasionally the patient can feel something slide around inside the knee. This injury requires medical attention.

Jumper's Knee. The tendon at the lower edge of the patella (kneecap) can be stretched and/or torn by repeated jumping. This is an overuse type problem, and one usually finds a series of microscopic tears rather than a single large tear. There will be marked point tenderness at the lower edge of the kneecap, and prolonged sitting with the knee bent will cause aching. The symptoms are aggravated by increased jumping. A program of rest, ice, massage, and anti-inflammatory medications is usually prescribed. Rest treatment is considerably more effective when initiated during the early onset of symptoms. If untreated, this problem is more likely to become chronic, and occasionally surgery is necessary.

Loose Bodies. Occasionally a fragment of bone or cartilage from the inside of the knee will break loose, and begin rolling around inside the joint.

These are known as "loose bodies". The patient can perceive this moving around, and occasionally can feel it with the fingers. When it is grasped, the loose body will suddenly squirt away. Loose bodies generally require surgical removal.

Chondromalacia Patella. The surface on the articular (joint) side of the patella is occasionally roughened. Symptoms usually include pain when climbing and descending stairs, hill, or ramps, and aching pain with prolonged sitting with the knee flexed. Running and jumping also cause increased pain. There is seldom swelling, and treatment generally consists of a specific exercise program to strengthen the thigh muscles. Treatment programs usually alleviate rather than eliminate symptoms.

Osgood-Schlatter's Disease. Eleven to fourteen year-old boys who run and jump excessively may irritate the growth plate at the insertion of the patellar tendon (below the kneecap). All of the powerful quadriceps muscles insert onto the tibia through the patellar tendon. Prior to completion of growth, this tendon inserts onto bone which is separated from the shaft of the tibia by a cartilage growth plate. This cartilage is unable to withstand the repeated abuse of excessive jumping, especially on hard surfaces. The cartilage growth plate becomes inflamed, and extremely painful. The pain is generally worsens with increased activity, and treatment consists of rest and anti-inflammatory medications. Although the symptoms generally disappear when growth is completed, this can be an extremely frustrating problem for active adolescents, and should be referred to a physician.

Ankle and Lower Leg Injuries

Sprains. The most common injury to the ankle is a sprain of its supporting ligaments. If the patient has tenderness directly over the bone, one must suspect a fracture, and x-rays are required. Ankle sprains are somewhat uncommon in young children. If massive swelling and discoloration or tenderness over the bone are present, medical consultation is recommended. Immediate care of ankle sprains consists of rest, ice, compression, elevation, and immobilization. Ankle sprains are best treated by rest (may require nonweight bearing on crutches or casting) until the symptoms subside. Trying to "walk off" a sprain is counterproductive in that additional tissue injury may occur. When the athlete is able to resume weight bearing, the ankle should be supported with tape or a functional brace until swelling, tenderness, and disability have subsided.

Shin Splints. Shin splints are one of the overuse syndromes, and appear along the medial (inside) of the tibia (shin bone). The symptoms will usually increase with activity, especially running and jumping on hard surfaces. There is seldom swelling or discoloration. If numbness, tingling, or swelling of the foot is present, prompt medical consultation is advised. Likewise, if the pain persists after a period of rest, medical consultation to rule out a stress fracture is recommended. Shin splints are often treated effectively with rest, anti-inflammatory medications, and arch supports. Ice and/or heat may also prove helpful in reducing inflammation and pain resulting from shin splints.

Foot Injuries

Stone Bruises. Jumping athletes may bruise the heel bone, or the fat pad immediately under the heel when the heel repeatedly strikes a hard surface. Heel cups and padded insoles are usually effective in diminishing symptoms.

Stress Fractures. Stress fractures are those fractures which occur from repeated small stresses rather than a single major injury. Stress fractures are commonly seen in the metatarsals (foot bones), and are often caused by increasing activity too quickly. The pain often begins three to four weeks after the start of an intensive training program, and there is point tenderness over the stress fracture site. Rest until the fracture heals, and then a wiser conditioning program are recommended treatments. Suspected stress fractures must be referred to a physician for evaluation and care.

Appendix A

Glossary

Aerobic - Literally, "with oxygen"; often used to refer to cardiovascular or cardiorespiratory fitness, as in aerobic fitness.

Anorexia nervosa - An eating disorder characterized by an abnormal preoccupation with being or becoming thin, which if untreated may result in serious illness and/or death.

Arrythmia - A variation from the normal rhythm of the heart beat.

Avulsion - (Musculoskeletal) A condition characterized by a tendon or ligament being forcefully pulled away from its bony attachment; (Dental) Displacement of a tooth from its socket.

Bulimia - An eating disorder characterized by an abnormal fear of gaining weight and an addiction to purging (vomiting or using strong laxatives) food in an attempt to lose/maintain weight; often called bulimia nervosa or bulimarexia.

Cardiorespiratory - Having to do with the heart, blood vessels, blood, lungs, and breathing passages; often used to refer to aerobic fitness, as in cardiorespiratory fitness.

Cardiovascular - Having to do with the heart, blood vessels, and blood; often used to refer to aerobic fitness, as in cardiovascular fitness.

Concussion - A loss of consciousness or other normal function, either temporary or prolonged, resulting from a blow or shock to the head.

Contusion - A bruise-type injury resulting from a blow to soft tissue by a blunt instrument.

Crepitation - Grating, grinding, or popping sound, often indicative of fractured bone ends rubbing together.

Cyanosis - A bluish discoloration of the skin resulting from a lack of oxygen.

Dislocation - A condition in which adjacent bones are completely separated from their normal joint relationship.

Diuretic - An agent that promotes urine secretion.

Epiphyseal plate - A specialized area of cartilage which exists in the growth areas (usually near the ends) of long bones; often called the "growth plate".

Epiphysis - The enlarged area at one or both ends of long bones.

Ergogenic aid - Anything used by an athletic in an attempt to enhance performance.

Esophagus - The tube-like structure connecting the mouth and stomach, through which food passes.

Extrusion - A pushing out as with an eye which has been extruded from its socket.

Femoral - Having to do with the thigh or femur, the large thigh bone.

Fracture - A crack or break in a bone.

Hamstrings - The muscle group which makes up the back portion of the thigh.

Hematologic - Having to do with the blood.

Hematoma - A pool or collection of blood within a tissue mass, often associated with a contusion.

Hematuria - The presence of blood in the urine.

Hemochromatosis - A disorder in which excess iron is deposited in the tissue.

Hypertension - Chronic high blood pressure.

Hypoxia - A condition in which there is a lack of sufficient oxygen in the body tissues.

...itis - A suffix which means an inflammation as in bursitis (an inflammation of bursa tissue) and tendinitis (an inflammation of tendon tissue).

Ligament - A tough band of tissue which binds bones together at joint sites to prevent excessive or abnormal movement.

Litigation - The legal process by which lawsuits are tried and resolved.

Marathon - A competitive foot race covering a distance of twenty-six miles, three hundred eighty-five yards.

Mononucleosis - An infectious viral condition, often characterized by fever, sore throat, and a general unwell feeling.

Myopia - Nearsightedness.

Myositis Ossificans - Calcium deposit within a muscle, usually caused by repeated contusions.

Ossification - The process by which the bones are formed.

Ostomy - An artificial body opening created by surgery, as with a colostomy.

Pathogenic - Health-threatening or disease-causing.

Periosteum - The outer covering or surface of a bone.

Peritoneum - The membrane which lines the walls of the abdominal and pelvic cavities.

Pseudonephritis - A common condition in athletes in which the presence of blood and other sediment in the urine gives a false indication of kidney disease; usually subsides with a reduction in physical activity.

Quadriceps - The muscle group which makes up the front portion of the thigh.

Retina - The innermost lining of the eye on which visual images are focused.

Respiratory - Having to do with the lungs and breathing passages.

Sinus bradycardia - A slowness of the heart rate, characterized by a pulse rate of less than 60 beats per minute.

Sprain - A stretch/tear injury to a ligament.

Strain - A stretch/tear injury to a muscle and/or tendon.

Subluxation - A condition in which adjacent bones are partially separated from their normal joint relationship.

Tendinitis - Inflammation of a tendon or tissue surrounding the tendon.

Tendon - A tough band of tissue which is the fibrous extension of a muscle, and attaches the muscle to bone.

Appendix B
Athletic Training Kit And Field Equipment

The kit should be large enough to carry enough supplies to administer first aid treatment to an athlete. The kit should also be large enough so the supplies can be easily reached Above all, the kit must always be kept neat and clean, emphasizing a professional appearance.

Apparatus:
Bandage Scissors
Tongue Forceps
Oral Screw
Plastic Airway
Nail Clippers
Tweezers
Small Scissors (pointed)
Thermometer (oral)
Safety Pins
Mirror (contact lens)
Pin Light (small flashlight)
Callus File
Tongue Blades
Cottom Tip Applicators
Plastic Bags (ice)
Latex gloves

Cotton/Gauze
Gauze Pads, sterile (3x3, 4x4)
Gauze Pads, non-stick
Gauze Roll
Stretch Gauze
Slings
Absorbent Cotton
Tampons (small)

Ointments
Skin Lubricant or Vaseline
Bacitracin
Triple Antibiotic Ointment
First Aid Cream
Antifungal Ointment
Vitamin A & D Ointment
Zinc Oxide Ointment

Solutions (Liquids)
Alcohol (2-4oz.)
Germicide-Fungicidel Liquid
Athletic Soap
Hydrogen Peroxide (4-6 oz.)
Eye Wash w/Cup

Bandaging Items
Elastic·Wraps (2", 4", 6")
Butterfly Closures (medium)
  or Steri-Strips
Adhesive Foam (1/8")
Band Aids (various sizes)
Adhesive Tape (1/2", 1", 1"')
Elastic Tape (2", 3")

Items To Be Found On Or Near Practice/Event Area
Ice Bags (disposable)
Water Containers (plenty of water)
Stretcher
Backboard
Crutches
Inflatable Air Splints (set)
Pad Bag (assortment of protective pads, wraps, foam rubber, etc.)
Tool Kit (pliers, screwdrivers, bolt cutters, pocket knife, etc.)
Clean Towels
Bleach (for bleach/water solution for blood clean-up)

Sports Medicine Program, North Carolina Department of Public Instruction, Raleigh, North Carolina. Modified and reprinted with permission.

Appendix C
Sample Forms

Athlete's Medical Form

This Section To Be Completed By Parent(s):

Name_____
        (Last)   (First)   (Middle)

S.S.#_____ Birth Date_____

Sex _____ Sport_____

Permanent Address: _____
                              (Street)

_____
        (City)   (State)   (Zip)

Phone (____) _____

PERSON TO BE NOTIFIED IN CASE OF EMERGENCY:

Name_____

Relationship_____

Address_____Phone (____)_____

PARENTS' INFORMATION:

Father's Full Name_____   Living? Yes___ No___

Mother's Full Name_____   Living? Yes___ No___

Parents' Address_____
                              (Street)

_____
        (City)   (State)   (Zip)

Phone: (Father's Home) _____ (Mother's Home) _____

(Father's Work) _____ (Mother's Work) _____

PARENT'S MEDICAL INSURANCE INFORMATION:

Insurance Company_____

Policy Number_____

Insurance Company's Address_____

Family Physician's Name_____

Family Physician's Address_____

This Section To Be Completed By Parent(s):
MEDICAL HISTORY: *All questions must be answered fully.*

		Yes	No	If yes, when?

1. Immunizations
a. Has your child been immunized against
measles, mumps, rubella, & polio? ___ ___ _____
b. Has your child ever had a positive TB test? ___ ___ _____
c. Has your child had a tetanus shot
in the last 10 years? ___ ___ _____

2. Head injury or concussion? ___ ___ _____

3. Eyes
a. Does your child have the absence of one eye? ___ ___ _____
b. Does your child wear glasses? ___ ___ _____
c. Does your child wear contact lenses? ___ ___ _____

4. Nose
a. Has your child's nose ever been broken? ___ ___ _____
b. Does your child have frequent nose bleeds? ___ ___ _____

5. Does your child have, or has he/she ever had any
of the following: (If yes, explain)

a. Dizzy spells, fainting, seizures ___ ___ _____
b. High blood pressure ___ ___ _____
c. Bleeding disorder ___ ___ _____
d. Allergies (food, drugs, or pollen) ___ ___ _____
e. Allergic reactions ___ ___ _____
f. Asthma ___ ___ _____
g. Bronchitis ___ ___ _____
h. Diabetes ___ ___ _____
i. Hernia (rupture) ___ ___ _____
j. Kidney disease ___ ___ _____
k. Appendicitis (Did you have surgery? Y / N) ___ ___ _____
l. Epilepsy ___ ___ _____
m. Jaundice or hepatitis ___ ___ _____
n. Polio ___ ___ _____
o. Frequent headaches (migraine?) ___ ___ _____
p. Infectious mononucleosis ___ ___ _____
q. Venereal disease ___ ___ _____
r. Rheumatic fever ___ ___ _____
s. Scarlet fever ___ ___ _____
t. Heart murmur ___ ___ _____
u. Loss of paired organ (kidney, eye, etc.) ___ ___ _____
v. Digestive ulcer ___ ___ _____
w. Heat cramps or heat exhaustion ___ ___ _____
x. Other _____

	Yes	No	If yes, when?

6. Musculoskeletal

a. Has your child ever dislocated a joint? ___ ___ _____
   1. If yes, which joint? _____
   2. Has it occurred more than once? ___ ___

b. Has your child ever injured his/her back? ___ ___ _____
   (If yes, explain) _____

c. Does your child have a spinal defect
   that has been present since birth? ___ ___

d. Has your child ever had a knee injury? ___ ___ _____
   1. Was surgery performed? (If yes, ___ ___ _____
     explain) _____
   2. Is he/she required to wear a brace? ___ ___

e. Has your child ever had an ankle sprain? ___ ___ _____
   1. Was surgery performed? ___ ___ _____
   2. Was the ankle casted? ___ ___
   3. Does his/her ankle require taping or
     other support? ___ ___

f. Has your child ever had a fracture? ___ ___ _____
   (If yes, where?) _____

g. Has your child ever developed myositis
   ossificans (calcium deposit)? ___ ___ _____
   1. If yes, where? _____
   2. Was surgery performed? ___ ___ _____

h. Has your child ever had surgery for any
   condition other than mentioned above? ___ ___ _____
   (If yes, explain) _____

7. Since his/her last exam, has your child seen a
   physician for any condition or has it been
   recommended that he/she see one? ___ ___ _____
   (Please explain)_____
_____
_____

     I hereby certify that my child has no known congenital or preexisting medical condition other than those identified above.

Parent's Signature_____ Date_____

This Section To Be Completed By A Physician:

MEDICAL EXAMINATION:

Height _____ Weight _____ Heart Rate _____ Blood Pressure _____

Vision (Snelling Chart): OS ____ OD ____ OU ____ Glasses? ___ Contacts? ___

	OK	Problem	Comment
Eyes	___	___	_____
Ears, nose, throat	___	___	_____
Head and neck	___	___	_____
Skin and scalp	___	___	_____
Lymphatics	___	___	_____
Thorax	___	___	_____
Lungs	___	___	_____
Heart	___	___	_____
Abdomen	___	___	_____
Hernia	___	___	_____
Genitalia	___	___	_____
Neurologic	___	___	_____
Shoulders	___	___	_____
Elbows	___	___	_____
Hands/wrists	___	___	_____
Back	___	___	_____
Knees	___	___	_____
Ankles	___	___	_____
Feet	___	___	_____

LAB TESTS

Urine Chemstrip 9: Leukocytes _____ Urine appearance: _____

Nitrite _____

Protein _____ Urine SpGr: _____

Glucose _____

Ketones _____ HCT: _____

Urobilinogen _____

Bilirubin _____ LMP: _____

Blood _____

pH _____ LPS: _____

PHYSICIAN EVALUATION:

____ No athletic participation _____

____ Limited athletic participation _____

____ Clearance withheld until _____

____ Full, unlimited athletic paticipation

Comments: _____

Physician's Signature _____ Date _____

Athletic Injury Report

REPORT FROM COACH/WORKER TO PHYSICIAN:

Name _____ Sport _____

Date of Report _____ Date of Injury _____

Person Completing Report _____

(Title) _____ (Phone) _____

Body Part Injured _____

Mechanism of Injury (How? What Happened?) _____
_____

Physical Findings _____
_____

Tentative Evaluation _____
_____

Immediate Care _____

Comments _____
_____

Follow Up:

_____ Physician Visit and/or X-rays Recommended on _____

_____ Physician Visit Not Recommended at This Time

_____   _____
(Parent's Signature)   (Coach's/Worker's Signature)

REPORT FROM PHYSICIAN TO COACH/WORKER:

Name _____ Sport _____

Diagnosis _____

Treatment Recommendations _____
_____

Copy of Specific Program Attached?   Yes _____   No _____

Estimated Time Out of Activity _____

Follow Up:

_____ Must see me/another physician prior to return to practice
and/or competition.

_____ May return to practice and/or competition immediately with
the following restrictions: _____
_____

_____ May return to practice and/or competition immediately with
no restrictions.

Comments _____

_____
(Physician's Signature)

_____   _____
(Date)   (Phone)

97

Appendix D

Common Drugs of Abuse

Drug	Other Name	Trade or Dangers	Effects	Physical Dependence	Psychological Dependence
STIMULANTS:					
Amphetamines	Biphetamine, Declobase, Desoxyn, Dexedrine, etc.	Paranoia, sexual impotence, death by O.D.	Increased alertness, excitation, euphoria	Possible	Yes
Cocaine*	Coke, flake snow	Nasal damage, toxic psychosis,	increased HR and BP, loss depression,	Possible	Yes
Cocaine hydrocholoride*	Crack	tremors, death	insomnia by O.D.	of appetite, Possible	Yes
DEPRESSANTS:					
Barbiturates	Phenobarbital, Secobarbital, Butisol, etc.	Blurred vision, nausea, seizures, death by O.D.	Disorientation, slurred speech, drunken behavior without odor	Yes	Yes
Methaqualone	Quaalude, Optimil, etc.	Nausea, seizures, death	of alcohol	Yes	Yes
Benzodiazepines	Valium, Librium, Dalmane, etc.	Hangover, menstrual problems death		Yes Yes	Yes Yes
HALLUCINOGENS:					
Marijuana	Pot, Acapulco gold, grass, etc.	Lung damage Reproductive re sperm and	Illusions, hallucinations, poor perception	?	Yes
Hashish and Hashish oil	Hash, Hash oil	ovulation, poor motor skill	of time and distance	?	Yes
Phencyclidine	PCP, Angel dust, etc.	Delerium, violent behavior		? ?	Yes Yes
LSD	Acid, microdot, etc.	Depression, physical exhaustion after use,		No	?
Mescaline and Peyote	Mesc, buttons, cactus, etc.	psychosis, exaggerated body distortion,		No	?
Amphetamine variants (Designer drugs)	2,5 DNA, DOP, STP, MDMA, DOM, etc.	fear of death, flashbacks, adverse drug reactions,		?	?
Other hallucinogens	DMT, DET, Ibogaine psilocybin, etc.	paranoia		No	?

Drug	Other Name	Trade or Dangers	Effects	Physical Dependence	Psychological Dependence
NARCOTICS:					
Opium	Dover's powder Paregoric, etc.	Respiratory and circulatory depression,	Euphoria, drowsiness, respiratory	Yes	Yes
Morphine	Morphine, Pectoral syrup etc.	dizziness, sweating, dry mouth, lowered	depression constricted pupils, nausea	Yes	Yes
Codeine	Empirin compound with Robitussin A-C, etc.	sex drive complications from injection		Yes	Yes
Heroin	Horse, smack, etc.	Same as above		Yes	Yes
Hydromorphone	Dilaudid	Same as above		Yes	Yes
Neperidine	Demerol, Pethadol, etc.	Same as above		Yes	Yes
Methadone	Dolophine, Methadose, etc.	Same as above		Yes	Yes
INHALANTS:					
Anesthetic gases	Petroleum products, solvents, aerosols	Head ache, nausea, nasal damage, bone marrow, liver,	Intoxication excitation, disorientation, aggression	No	Possible
Vasodilators (amyl nitrite, butyl nitrite)	Petroleum products, solvents, aerosols	heart, kidney and CNS damage	hallucination, variable effects	No	Possible
Anabolic steroids	Roids, juice etc.	Liver, heart, and blood problems cancer, agression, ("Roid rage")	Increased muscle mass under certain conditions	?	Possible

*Cocaine is designated a narcotic under the Controlled Substances Act.

Appendix E

Selected Stretching Exercises

1. Warm the muscles prior to stretching by jogging easily or doing light calisthenics.

2. Place the muscles in the stretch position shown, and hold that position for 30 to 45 seconds.

3. Do not bounce or jerk the muscles during stretching.

4. Do not stretch to the point of pain, but rather until slight tension is felt.

5. Always stretch both arms, both legs, both sides, etc.

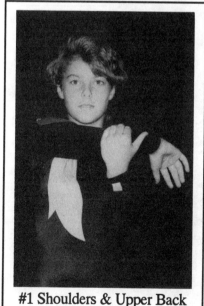

#1 Shoulders & Upper Back

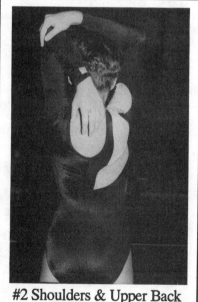

#2 Shoulders & Upper Back

Photos by: Bob Stone, Greenwood, South Carolina

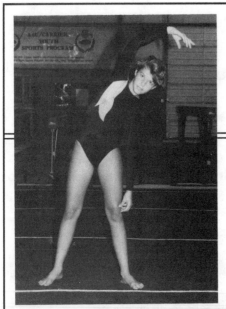

#3 Trunk Muscles

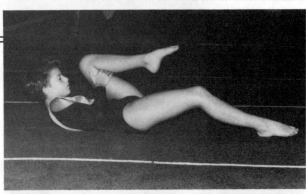

#4 Lower Back,
Hips, and
Hamstrings

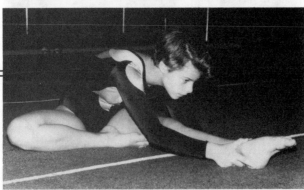

#5 Hamstrings

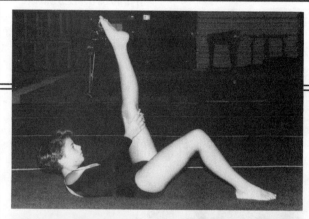

#6 Hamstrings

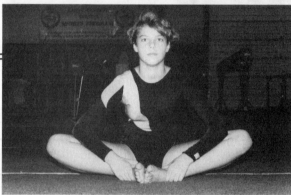

#7 Groin Muscles

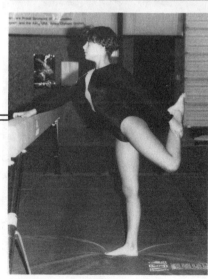

#8 Quadriceps

Photos by: Bob Stone,
Greenwood, South Carolina

*Photos by: Bob Stone,
Greenwood, South Carolina*

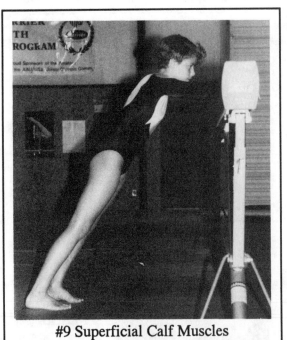

#9 Superficial Calf Muscles

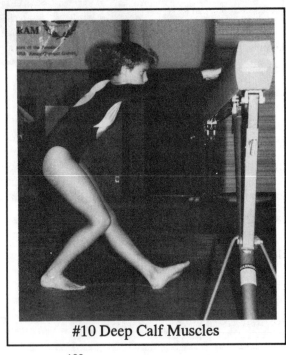

#10 Deep Calf Muscles

Index

Index, *continued*